INTEGRATED HEALTH CARE:

Case Studies

by

Dean C. Coddington
and
Barbara J. Bendrick

Center for Research in Ambulatory Health Care Administration (CRAHCA) publications are intended to provide current and accurate information and are designed to assist readers in becoming more familiar with the subject matter covered. CRAHCA published *Integrated Health Care: Case Studies* for a general audience. Such publications are distributed with the understanding that CRAHCA does not render any legal, accounting or other professional advice that may be construed as specifically applicable to individual situations. No representations or warranties are made concerning the application of legal or other principles discussed by the authors to any specific fact situation, nor is any prediction made concerning how any particular judge, government official or other person who will interpret or apply such principles. Specific factual situations should be discussed with professional advisers.

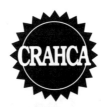

TABLE OF CONTENTS

INTRODUCTION

This is the companion volume to *Integrated Health Care: Reorganizing the Physician, Hospital and Health Plan Relationship* published by the Center for Research in Ambulatory Health Care Administration (CRAHCA).

The nine case studies included in this volume were an important part of the database used in preparing Volume I.* Part B of Volume I, in particular, relies heavily on a cross-sectional analysis of what was learned from the case studies.

The introduction to Part B of Volume I identifies the factors considered in selecting the case study organizations. Exhibit A is a map showing the location of each participating organization.

The case studies contained in this book are descriptive and presented in a format intended to facilitate discussion and training. The written case studies provide more detailed information about each of the participating integrated health care systems than it was possible to present in Volume I.

Each of the case studies involved initial collection of information, a two to three-day field visit, follow-up interviews and data collection, and the preparation of the written case study. The case studies were reviewed by representatives of each of the participating organizations and approved for publication.

The case studies are presented in the order in which they were prepared. The month on the title page of each case study reflects when the field work was completed, and the case studies were current as of that point in time. Given the dynamics of the health care industry, and integrated health care systems in particular, there have been subsequent changes in the status of most of these organizations. Nevertheless, the case studies should be useful to individuals desiring in-depth information about how organizations have progressed toward becoming more fully-integrated health care systems.

The title page for each case study identifies the participants and their positions in the organization. We appreciate the willingness of these individuals to share their time, experience and insights for the benefit of others who desire to learn more about what it takes to move along the path toward becoming a more fully integrated health care system.

---

* One of the organizations analyzed and included in Volume I, Montana Associated Physicians Inc. and Saint Vincent Hospital, declined permission to include its case study in this volume.

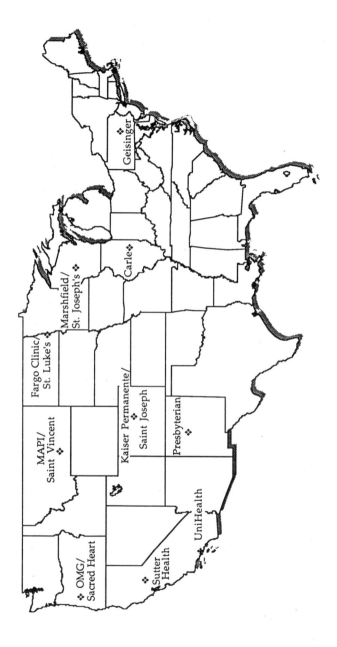

EXHIBIT A.
Location of Case Study Organizations

THE AUTHORS

Dean C. Coddington is a founder of BBC Research & Consulting, located in Denver, Colorado. He received his BS degree (1954) from South Dakota State University in civil engineering and his MBA degree (1959) from the Harvard Business School.

Coddington has written numerous articles, including four published in the *Harvard Business Review*. He is co-author of two previous books: *Market-Driven Strategies in Health Care* (1987) and *The Crisis in Health Care: Costs, Choices and Strategies* (1990). His research and consulting focuses on the factors driving health care costs, market research, economic feasibility studies and strategic planning for health care organizations.

From 1959 to 1970, Coddington worked as a research economist with the University of Denver's Research Institute. He is also past chairman of the board of trustees of Swedish Medical Center, Englewood, Colorado.

Barbara J. Bendrick joined BBC as an associate in 1992. She received her BS degree (1988) from Wright State University in finance and her MBA degree (1992) from the University of Florida.

Bendrick has been involved in a number of health care assignments since joining BBC, including the development of a physician-hospital organization, financial modeling for an HMO, and the merger of a medical group and hospital.

Between 1988 and 1992, Bendrick worked as a financial analyst for a financial planning firm in Columbus, Ohio, a finance intern for BellSouth Advertising & Publishing and a teaching assistant at the University of Florida.

BBC Research & Consulting was established in 1970 to provide economic and policy analysis to clients in a variety of industries. BBC's health care practice focuses on strategic planning, financial feasibility assessments and market analyses for hospitals, medical groups and health plans throughout the country.

ABOUT THE CENTER FOR RESEARCH IN AMBULATORY HEALTH CARE ADMINISTRATION AND THE MEDICAL GROUP MANAGEMENT ASSOCIATION

The Center for Research in Ambulatory Health Care Administration (CRAHCA), established in 1973, is a section 501(c)(3) tax-exempt charitable organization as defined by the Internal Revenue Code. The purpose of CRAHCA is to improve ambulatory health care in general and group practice in particular through better administration. Its work focuses on new and innovative publications; education, research, and data services; and demonstration programs. The Center for Research in Ambulatory Health Care Administration is the research arm of the Medical Group Management Association (MGMA).

Founded in 1926, the Medical Group Management Association today comprises over 14,700 members and 5,900 medical groups involving about 111,000 physicians. It is the oldest and largest membership organization representing group practice administration. MGMA serves its individual and organizational members and their patients, and promotes the group practice of medicine as an effective form of health care delivery.

The relationships between medical groups, hospitals, and health plans are an important area of interest to CRAHCA. The more integrated the relationships among the three "legs of the stool", the greater the challenge is for CRAHCA to study ambulatory care in the new evolving organizational relationships in which physicians and group practices play an important role. These changes are posing significant challenges to CRAHCA and MGMA to change definitions as the environment is changing and to refocus its research agenda to meet the needs of these integrating organizations. In addition, CRAHCA has a mission to educate the ambulatory health care community on the changing environments.

To meet both of these objectives, CRAHCA is pleased to publish the book *Integrated Health Care: Case Studies* as a very important and timely piece of work. Funding was provided from the CRAHCA Research and Development Fund. These funds were utilized to support the site visits and other data collection efforts of the authors, and in providing additional resources to them to analyze their findings, adding significantly to the value of this book.

We want to thank the organizations that shared their experience with the authors. They did this understanding the importance of sharing their learning experiences with the health care community, in general, and the MGMA membership in particular. It was important to focus the research on operating integrated health care systems as opposed to those that are in the nascent stages. The reader thus gets a perspective on the sets of circumstances and conditions important to an integrated organization.

We would like to thank the authors for taking the initiative to develop the idea for this text and for their interest and willingness in working with CRAHCA to publish it.

Case Study #1

PRESBYTERIAN
HEALTHCARE SERVICES
Albuquerque, New Mexico

— Persons Contacted —

Richard Barr, President, Presbyterian Healthcare Services
Andrew Horvath, MD, Chairman, Network Board
John Koster, MD, former Vice President, Network Development
William Daugherty, MD, Medical Director of Primary Care
Marvin Feit, Chief Information Officer, Presbyterian Healthcare Services
Kim Hedrick, Vice President, Network Development
David Hildebrand, Clinical Project Coordinator, Quality Support Services
Neil Kaminsky, MD, Network Managed Care Director, HealthPlus
Peter Snow, Vice President, Planning & Managed Care
Stephen Spare, MD, Chairman, Physician Management Board

February, 1993

EXHIBIT A
Location of Albuquerque, New Mexico

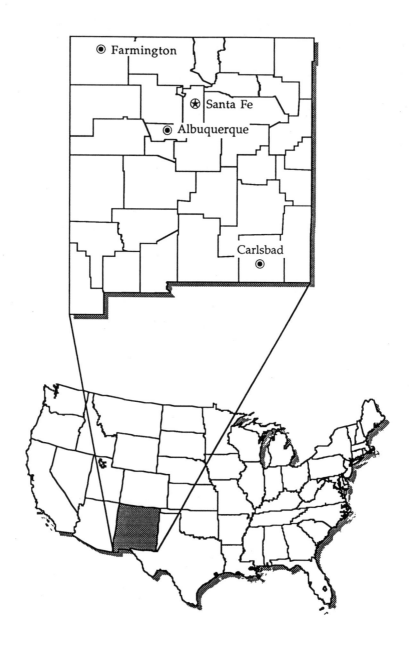

PRESBYTERIAN HEALTHCARE SERVICES
Albuquerque, New Mexico

During our briefing with Richard Barr, President of Presbyterian Healthcare Services (PHS), he told us, "We are trying to reinvent the way we deliver health care in Albuquerque and New Mexico." This case study describes how this was being accomplished as of early 1993.

Barr used the term "organized care" to describe PHS and the Network. He defined this type of care as a "regional organization of health care providers who come together voluntarily to manage the care of patients and accept risk for the care of a defined population over time."

The Albuquerque Health Care Marketplace

The population of the Albuquerque Metropolitan Area was 612,000 in early 1993. Exhibit A shows the location of PHS sites throughout the State of New Mexico.

For the State as a whole, an estimated 28 percent of the population was uninsured. In Albuquerque, the percentage of uninsured was estimated to be 20 percent.

Health plan coverage patterns. The Albuquerque health care marketplace has been dominated by managed care, especially health maintenance organizations (HMOs). Between 1988 and early 1993, there was an 88 percent increase in HMO penetration of the insured population; managed care covered 78 percent by 1993. The growth in health plan enrollment, primarily HMOs, in Albuquerque between 1984 and 1988 is shown in Exhibit B.

In mid-1992, five HMOs had 263,000 members. The largest was CIGNA-Lovelace with 136,500, followed by HealthPlus (the Presbyterian health plan) with 54,000 members, Foundation Health Plan (FHP) with 33,000 members, QualMed (24,000) and HMO New Mexico (Blue Cross and Blue Shield) at 15,000. PHS and its physicians were the exclusive provider for this latter plan and provided about 60 percent of the care for QualMed subscribers until PHS canceled the hospital contract with QualMed in 1993.

Exhibit B.

HEALTH PLAN ENROLLMENT

Plan	1988	1989	1990	1991	6/92
Lovelace	100,145	111,616	119,569	125,735	136,537
Health Plus					
HMO	30,607	27,580	29,678	35,004	40,819
PPO	6,240	8,185	7,881	6,101	6,056
SPN				6,400	7,170
Subtotal	36,847	35,765	37,559	47,505	54,045
FHP					
Seniors	8,678	10,280	12,589	13,108	18,206
Commercial	10,800	12,665	15,620	15,906	14,930
Subtotal	19,478	22,945	28,209	29,014	33,136
Qual-Med	24,269	20,790	19,276	22,923	24,044
HMO NM	8,346	10,548	11,671	12,208	14,956
Total	189,085	201,664	216,264	238,395	262,718

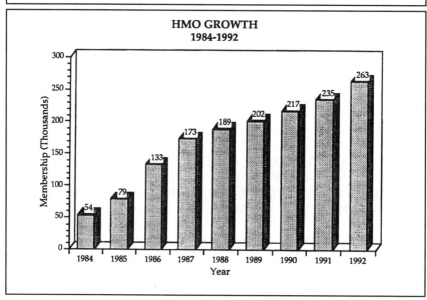

HMO GROWTH
1984-1992

Source: Presbyterian Healthcare Services, 1993.

Participation in preferred provider organizations (PPOs) in Albuquerque was approximately 88,000 in mid-1992.

Competition. When driving the Albuquerque freeways, a visitor is struck by the large number of billboards advertising local hospital systems and health plans, an indicator of the competitive nature of the local health care market.

There were four health care systems (eight hospitals and 1,500 physicians) operating in Albuquerque in early 1993:

- *CIGNA-Lovelace.* Established in 1972, Lovelace includes a multispecialty clinic, a group practice HMO, and a 197-bed hospital. The system provides services in 13 patient care facilities in Albuquerque, Santa Fe and Las Cruces. There were 350 physicians in the multispecialty group practice and clinics.

  Membership in the health plan totaled approximately 120,000 (the plan lost the State of New Mexico contract in early 1993 and dropped from nearly 140,000 members in mid-1992). Over 60 percent of Lovelace's revenues come from prepaid premiums.

- *University of New Mexico.* University Medical Center is a 309-bed tertiary care facility with 400 employed physicians. Many of its patients are on Medicaid or are uninsured, and it receives a state tax subsidy.

- *St. Joseph Healthcare System.* This system has three hospitals with 500 beds in Albuquerque. There are approximately 500 physicians on the medical staff of its three hospitals. St. Joseph and its physicians are the delivery network for FHP. Among specialists, there is substantial overlap between St. Joseph's and Presbyterian's hospitals.

- *Presbyterian Healthcare System (PHS).* PHS has three acute care hospitals in Albuquerque (total of 628 beds) and 13 hospitals in smaller communities throughout New Mexico and Colorado. The medical staff in Albuquerque numbers 600, of which 120 are primary care physicians. HealthPlus, the organization's health plan, had 54,000 members as of early 1993, up substantially from mid-1992. PHS operated 11 primary care practice locations throughout the Albuquerque area.

According to Richard Barr, Presbyterian's three Albuquerque hospitals have about 40 percent of the inpatient days in the metro area market. He also mentioned that nearly one-third of the hospitals' patients originate outside of Albuquerque. Exhibit C shows the location of Presbyterian's facilities in the Albuquerque area.

History of the Presbyterian Network

The origins of the formation of the Presbyterian Network date back to 1988 when a primary care task force, or alliance, was formed for the purpose of strengthening primary care at Presbyterian. At that time, 17 primary care physicians met to figure out how to organize. Several of these physicians were considering leaving private practice and going to work for Lovelace. Physicians expressed frustration over managed care, lower reimbursements and difficulties of managing a practice in a very competitive market. The main purpose of the alliance was to provide a forum for primary care physicians to discuss issues affecting their specialty.

In 1989, Andrew Horvath, MD, a pathologist on the Presbyterian medical staff, was asked to chair a task force to identify and assess issues relating to the future of physicians and the relationship between Presbyterian and its medical staff. This was called the Physician-Hospital Organization and Decision-M aking Task Force. During a briefing, Dr. Horvath said, "I agreed to accept this job, and thought it might take a couple of meetings. Here we are four years later and we have put in a huge amount of time." The task force included 11 physician leaders and four PHS system managers. Out of this task force, the Network Board was formed.

Dr. Horvath continued, "As a part of the Board's work, we went through an environmental assessment, a look ahead at the health care market in general with emphasis on Albuquerque. This made us realize that we were going to have to do something fast. We prepared a document, called the Network Development Report, and made a presentation to the PHS Board of Trustees concerning our ideas and recommendations. (The PHS Board is the community board of trustees which oversees the Presbyterian Health Services operations.) They told us to keep going." This then led to the proposal to form the Network Development Task Force which evolved into the Network Board (September 1990). The Task Force report proposed 12 strategic initiatives to link physician practices and Presbyterian hospitals into an integrated health care organization (the Network Board).

EXHIBIT C.
Location of Presbyterian's Family Healthcare Offices, Hospitals and Physician Practices, 1993

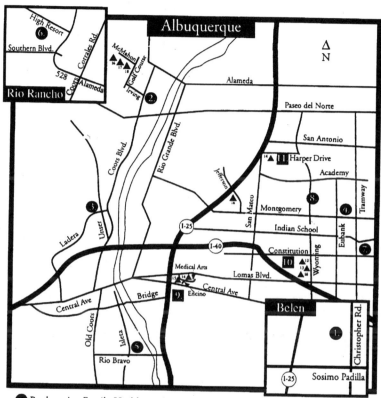

● Presbyterian Family Healthcare (PFH)

1. PFH - Belen
2. PFH - Coors (Future)
3. PFH - Ladera
4. PFH - Montgomery (Future)
5. PFH - Rio Bravo
6. PFH - Rio Rancho
7. PFH - Tramway (Future)
8. PFH - Wyoming

■ Hospitals

9. Presbyterian Hospital
10. Presbyterian Kaseman Hospital
11. Presbyterian Northside Hospital

▲ Physician Practices

12. Adult Health Care Specialists
13. New Mexico Arthritis Clinic
14. Albuquerque OB-GYN Specialists (2 Locations)
15. Albuquerque Endocrinology Consultants
16. Mesa Mental Health (3 Locations)
17. West Mesa Family Medicine
18. West Mesa Pediatric Associates

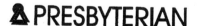
PRESBYTERIAN

Dr. Horvath described the process of selecting members for the Network Board. "We picked individuals who could think strategically, and put their own interests aside." He said that there were 60 volunteers, and a questionnaire and interview process was used to narrow the selection down to 11 physicians. This process took two months.

In looking back, Peter Snow, Vice President for Planning and Managed Care, and a member of the Presbyterian management team for a decade, noted that, "In the beginning, the primary motivation for forming the Network was defensive; it was in response to managed care growth and the aggressive moves of several of our competitors, especially Lovelace. It has since evolved to include the potential to improve the delivery of health care for payors and patients." Snow went on to point out that prior to 1988, managed care (with the exception of Lovelace) was not viewed as much of a threat since the provider panels (both physicians and hospitals) tended to be broad (many physicians and hospitals contracted with several health plans). "However, in 1988 this changed as health plans began to contract with single systems. This is when physicians and hospitals began to see the potential for significant losses of patients."

As an indication of the changes that have taken place at PHS since 1990, Richard Barr concluded, "I no longer think in terms of the system as hospitals; I think of it as the Network."

Network Mission Statement and Responsibilities

The Presbyterian Network mission statement says:

"The Network brings together physicians, PHS hospitals, and other health care services. The Network's purpose is to provide the highest value health care possible: both premier quality and cost-effective services required to sustain leadership in a highly competitive marketplace."

The primary responsibility, or "charge," for the Network Board included:

1.   Identification, assessment and selection of Network development initiatives.

2.   Recommendation of PHS investment in Network activities.

3.   Determination of physician participation in Network initiatives. This included criteria for selection of participants and the selection process.

4.   Monitoring of Network implementation plans.

5.   Strategic planning for PHS and its physicians.

On the last point, Dr. Horvath noted that PHS has had a strategic planning committee for many years, but the PHS Board made the decision to delegate this function to the Network Board. However, he emphasized that the PHS Board maintains the ultimate authority.

Extent of Integration at Presbyterian

The approach to participation in physician-hospital integration within Presbyterian is flexible. The range is from participation in normal medical staff activities, including quality assurance and marketing, to full economic integration (described later) and employment. Exhibit D demonstrates the conceptual approach to integration at PHS. To participate in the services and systems described in the four boxes to the right, a physician must be part of the Network.

Becoming Part of the Network

Application process. Initially, all members of the Presbyterian medical staff could apply for membership in the Network. The application process included a willingness to attend a two-hour meeting to be briefed on the Network (more than 50 such meetings have been held) and to complete a detailed questionnaire. The questionnaire includes, among other items, information on malpractice allegations and lawsuits, expression of a commitment to be actively involved in continuous quality improvement (CQI), and a commitment to attend quarterly general membership meetings relating to the Network. Physicians wishing to continue as members of the Network must apply for recredentialing every two years.

The Network Selection Committee, the group responsible for developing criteria and screening applicants, reports to the PHS Board. The committee is made up of four PHS board members, two PHS administrators, and two physicians (one primary care and one specialist). The composition of the committee — it emphasizes non-physician members — was designed to protect the Network from possible antitrust and restraint of trade problems.

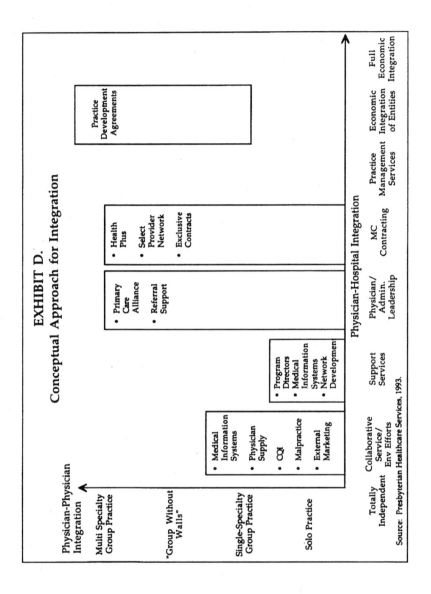

EXHIBIT D.
Conceptual Approach for Integration

Physician-Physician Integration

- Multi-Specialty Group Practice
- "Group Without Walls"
- Single-Specialty Group Practice
- Solo Practice

Practice Development Agreements

- Primary Care Alliance
- Referral Support

- Health Plus
- Select Provider Network
- Exclusive Contracts

- Program Directors
- Medical Information Systems
- Network Developmen

- Medical Information Systems
- Physician Supply
- CQI
- Malpractice
- External Marketing

Physician-Hospital Integration

Totally Independent — Collaborative Service/ Env Efforts — Support Services — Physician/ Admin. Leadership — MC Contracting — Practice Management Services — Economic Integration of Entities — Full Economic Integration

Source: Presbyterian Healthcare Services, 1993.

The selection questionnaire consists of questions divided into the following categories with scoring weighted heavily towards quality.

I. Total Quality = 60 Percent Weight

1. Clinical Quality
2. Cost Effectiveness
3. Patient Satisfaction
4. Reputation
5. Compatibility
6. Unique Capabilities

II. Affiliation = 40 Percent Weight

1. Percent of Hospital Utilization in Network
2. Referral Patterns within Network
3. Health Plan Usage

By early 1992, the Selection Committee had completed a nine-month review process leading to the selection of its initial group of physicians. Approximately 400 physicians applied for membership in the Network; 18 were rejected. John Koster, MD, and former Senior Vice President for Network Development, noted that the major part of the selection process involved physicians' deciding whether or not to apply for membership. "Over 200 physicians decided not to participate and did not complete the application process. This was the real screener — meaning that the application process itself caused some self-selection out of the Network due to the types of questions we are asking."

Physicians invited to be part of the Network, as a result of successfully meeting all selection criteria, signed a Network Affiliation Agreement. This is a binding contract that remains in effect until the physician decides to terminate the Agreement, violates the rules of the Network (e.g., not completing medical records in a timely manner, not attending meetings, not participating in CQI projects), or is not recredentialed in two years. All Network contracted activities will be treated as an addendum to the Network Affiliation Agreement (i.e., participation in the PHS Doctor Referral Service).

Benefits of Network to physicians. What are the benefits of Network affiliation (what is in it for me)? According to Dr. Horvath, some that are most important are:

- Ability to participate in quality programs (CQI and outcomes measurement) and to be marketed as the Network. Horvath emphasized, "If we don't make a major effort to improve our quality and measure our outcomes, we don't have a marketable product."

- Potential to be involved in a Practice Development Agreement (described later).

- Participation in family health care centers and a multispecialty clinic.

- Contracting opportunities. This refers to participation in direct contracts with payors and continuing involvement with HealthPlus.

- Practice management. This includes an array of services provided by PHS, including billing, collections and professional management.

- Information systems. This will be especially important in the future (see later discussion).

The Presbyterian Network and Medical Staff

Dr. Horvath contrasted the role of the PHS medical staff with that of the Network Board (see Exhibit E). He noted that the Network Board deals with economic and business issues, while the medical staff deals primarily with clinical and professional issues within the hospitals. "The term 'Network' may be too soft for the kind of business partnerships being entered into by PHS and certain physicians. This is definitely a business venture with strong economic incentives."

On the matter of membership in the Presbyterian Network, Dr. Horvath said it is important to understand that while the medical staff is generally open to all qualified physicians, Network participation is based on the needs of the Network. This, of course, relates to the success of the Network in building its primary care base and competing for managed care contracts. "This has been a difficult concept for physicians to understand, because when they entered into this relationship most thought of the Network as another PPO. Now that we are gaining market share, non-Network physicians find themselves on the outside of some contracts and that's frustrating."

EXHIBIT E.
Comparison of Responsibilities for Network Board
and PHS Medical Staff

	PHS MEDICAL STAFF EXECUTIVE COMMITTEE	**NETWORK BOARD**
1. PRINCIPAL ROLE OR PURPOSE	DEALS PRIMARILY WITH CLINICAL AND PROFESSIONAL ISSUES WITHIN THE HOSPITAL	• DEALS PRIMARILY WITH ECONOMIC AND BUSINESS ISSUES RELATED TO NETWORK STRATEGIC PLANNING
2. PRIMARY RESPONSIBILITIES	• CREDENTIALLING • QUALITY ASSURANCE • CONTINUING MEDICAL EDUCATION	• EVALUATE AND RECOMMEND INITIATIVES • MONITOR THE NETWORK IMPLEMENTATION PLAN
3. MEMBERSHIP	GENERALLY OPEN TO ALL QUALIFIED PHYSICIANS	PHYSICIAN PARTICIPATION BASED ON THE NEEDS OF THE NETWORK
4. REPORTING RELATIONSHIP	REPORTS DIRECTLY TO THE PHS BOARD OF DIRECTORS	REPORTS DIRECTLY TO THE PHS BOARD OF DIRECTORS

Source: Presbyterian Healthcare Services, 1993.

According to a number of physicians, there continues to be confusion concerning the role of the medical staff versus the role of the Network. However, as one physician noted: "It is impossible to organize a medical staff to accomplish anything related to new business development, managed care contracting, or working together with the hospital in the formation of an organized delivery system of the type needed to compete in this marketplace, and to be successful under health care reform."

Richard Barr said, "Our medical staff functions in the traditional manner. We are concerned about future physician medical staff leadership because most of the action is with the Network."

Governance of the Presbyterian Network

Exhibit F shows the organizational structure for the PHS Board, the Network Board, the Network Selection Committee, the PHS Medical Executive Committee and several formal committees of the Network Board.

PHS Board. This consists of 27 members who serve as the board for all Presbyterian hospitals. This board functions as the typical board of a multihospital system with emphasis on medical staff credentialing, assuring that the system has a strategic plan, approving the annual budget and capital expenditures, monitoring performance, and hiring the system CEO.

According to Barr, "The Network is not a legal entity; PHS is the legal entity."

Network Board. In place three years, the Network Board reports to the PHS Board. It is made up of 16 physicians (seven primary care physicians, nine medical specialists), two PHS administrators and one PHS Board member. The mission statement and responsibilities of this Board were discussed earlier.

Physician Management Board. The Physician Management Board reports to the Network Board, and its primary responsibility is to set policies for economically-integrated physicians (referred to as EIP's on Exhibit F). In early 1993, approximately 70 primary care physicians were economically integrated into the Network.

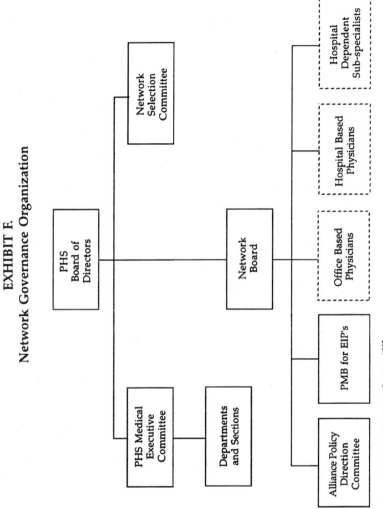

EXHIBIT F.
Network Governance Organization

Source: Presbyterian Healthcare Services, 1993.

The Physician Management Board has 15 voting members (14 physicians and one PHS administrator), and meets every two weeks. Practice managers, who are PHS employees are nonvoting members of the Physician Management Board. Physician members are elected by their respective medical groups; they are the lead physicians in each of these groups. Members are elected for two years, but they can be replaced by physicians in their medical practice. Members of this board are paid for their time at the rate of one-quarter of their normal compensation.

In talking with Stephen Spare, MD, Chairman of the Physician Management Board, we learned that the primary duties of the board include development of health plan products (e.g., a Medicare risk plan), contracting guidelines, participation in the Network budgeting process, evaluation of pension issues, physician compensation and performance evaluation and collaboration on Joint Commission on Accreditation of Healthcare Organizations (JCAHO) matters. (One of the by-products of economic integration of physicians has been the need for family health care sites to be part of the JCAHO accreditation process.)

Looking ahead, Dr. Spare expects this board to become involved in issues surrounding the incorporation of medical specialists into the Network. Another matter likely to become important in the future is how to handle relationships with physicians in the smaller communities outside of Albuquerque.

Other Network Board committees. In early 1993 there were four sub-boards or committees under the Network Board, including the Physician Management Board just described.

The sub-boards represent office-based physicians (dermatologists, ophthalmologists), hospital-based physicians (pathologists, anesthesiologists, radiologists, emergency medicine doctors), and hospital-dependent subspecialists (cardiologists, cardiovascular surgeons, general surgeons, urologists, orthopedic surgeons and others who are active users of the hospital).

The role of the sub-boards is to facilitate two-way communication between the Network Board and the physician members of the Network. Members of the boards were elected to two-year terms and the chair of each board is a voting member of the Network Board. The circular representation for all the boards is instrumental in facilitating accurate, timely communication.

HealthPlus Board. The insurance arm of the Network is represented by HealthPlus, Inc. The Board is made up of six physicians and three administrators who oversee the operations of a triple option health maintenance organization (HMO). HealthPlus offers PPO, indemnity, small group and Medicare-risk products. In early 1991, HealthPlus agreed to "rent" its provider panel directly to self-insured employers and other national PPOs through a product called Select Provider Network (SPN). An access fee for panel management, utilization review and/or claims processing options is typically charged for SPN.

Economic Integration and Financial Arrangements

This is one of the key aspects of physician-hospital integration at PHS. As noted earlier, 80 physicians were part of financial arrangements that tie them to PHS.

Practice Development Agreement (PDA). This agreement is the document that links physicians and PHS together into the integrated Network. According to Bill Daugherty, MD, Medical Director of Primary Care at PHS, the goals of the agreement are to:

- Align economic and market incentives for physicians and PHS.

- Free physicians from day-to-day operations so they can practice medicine.

- Create mechanisms to pursue market opportunities not available to physicians or hospitals individually.

- Share the risk of practice expansion and physician recruitment.

- Rationalize technology (make sure that the right amount of technology is available in the right locations).

Dr. Daugherty said, "The Practice Development Agreement can be thought of as a lease of the practice by PHS with a lease payment to the physician corporation. The level of the lease payment is based upon historical compensation and current year incentives." He noted that this agreement is similar to the contract between PHS and emergency medicine physicians.

The mechanics of the PDA include:

- All practice assets are leased by PHS from physician owners at fair market value. These include the building lease or mortgage payment, equipment leases and other practice-related debts.

- All non-physician employees of the practice become employees of PHS.

- A practice manager (PHS employee) reports to the Practice Management Division of PHS.

- A budget for the coming year is jointly developed by the practice and PHS, and this includes physician compensation.

Under the original PDA, there was a risk sharing agreement between physicians and PHS. If practice net income (after payment to physicians) exceeded the budget forecasts (which has since been revised to meet Medicare safe harbor laws) for the year, one-quarter of the surplus goes to PHS and three-quarters is divided among the physicians. However, the amount due physicians is added to their expected income for the following year; it is not paid out as a lump sum bonus.

Decision making under this new arrangement is as follows:

PHS	**Consensus**	**Physicians**
Personnel policies	Practice management	Patient care
Staff salaries	Equipment acquisition	Referrals to specialists
Supervision	Hours of service	and hospitals
	Staffing/office operations	
	Physician recruitment	
	Contracting	

Strengths of PDA. Dr. Daugherty summarized the positive aspects of the PDA as follows:

- Creates partnership approach
- Articulates the expectation of a long-term relationship
- Creates sense of security for both parties
- Improves physician productivity (in most cases)
- Creates ability to contract on behalf of physicians' professional corporation
- Improved benefits for physicians

Weaknesses of PDA. These include the perception among some physicians that those entering into a PDA have "sold out" to PHS, difficulty in accommodating income expectations of all physicians, and the difficulty of implementation for solo practitioners and small groups. On this latter point, Dr. Daugherty said, "It is virtually impossible for physicians to get together. It is easier for them to join with PHS; there seems to be less suspicion and more trust."

A physician perspective. Dr. Daugherty used his own practice as a case study of what can happen with economic integration. In 1989 his practice had 3.75 full-time equivalent physicians in one location on the west side of Albuquerque. The group participated in 10 managed care plans. Physician income had been stagnant for three years, and they were losing market share to Lovelace and FHP. "The truth of the matter is that our finances were on a month-to-month basis, and we never knew whether or not we would have anything to take home."

The decision to participate in economic integration with PHS was driven by a number of factors including the "obvious erosion of our financial base." Dr. Daugherty also cited the growing "hassle factor" of working with managed care, inability to recruit new physicians, insufficient funds to contribute to their pension plan, and a feeling that "we were losing control of our practice." He added, "We needed a bigger, tougher older brother, and we saw this in PHS."

Three and a half years later, this medical practice had grown to nine physicians in three locations in west Albuquerque, and it participated in 25 health plans. Dr. Daugherty said that once they signed the PDA, there was "an instant feeling of relief." Other factors were:

- Practice is stable
- Incomes have increased
- Retirement plan contributions are made
- Hassle factor is down

Dr. Daugherty added, "I think PHS has also benefited in terms of a major presence on the west side, it has added to the base of physicians in this area, and it has enhanced its credibility in terms of physician relations." He also mentioned that PHS's involvement has also increased the system's understanding of primary care medicine.

Looking ahead. Dr. Daugherty views the growing number of PDAs as the fundamental building block of the Network. He referred primarily to contracting and overall clinical/management relationships. He also believes that economic integration will pay off in terms of lower costs, improved effectiveness in the delivery of care, and increased physician productivity. He added, "There is the potential to aggregate PDA participants into larger groups."

Among the challenges facing his practice and PHS, Dr. Daugherty cited physician compensation for both primary care and specialists ("the market will drive this"), legal issues, the New Mexico gross receipts tax (it adds six percent to medical bills), symbolism versus reality in terms of the Network, and the "innies" vs. the "outies." He looks forward to achieving what he calls a seamless patient care system with documented quality results. He also hopes for improved primary care physician income and stability.

Presbyterian Involvement in Managed Care

Presbyterian's initial entry into managed care was with the formation of Mastercare, an IPA-model HMO, in 1972. According to Neil Kaminsky, MD, Network Managed Care Director, the HMO ran into utilization problems, dissatisfaction among physicians and patient migration in and out of the plan. "Even with these problems, the plan achieved a membership of 25,000."

Despite this growth, the HMO's board discontinued the plan in 1981. Two-thirds of the participants in Mastercare immediately enrolled in the Lovelace HMO. Dr. Kaminsky said, "This move to Lovelace was a shock to physicians at Presbyterian. We thought we had the loyalty of our patients. However, we found out that many of them liked the concept of an HMO better than they liked us."

A second generation HMO, called HealthPlus, was started in 1986. The plan was a joint venture between Presbyterian and St. Joseph, but St. Joseph sold its share to PHS in 1989. The physician provider network was originally an IPA, but according to Dr. Kaminsky, "This organization — the IPA — self destructed a few years ago. Now each physician contracts independently with the health plan."

HealthPlus grew to 54,000 members and over 400 businesses by 1993. While it mainly served Albuquerque, northern New Mexico and Socorro, the plan continued to expand statewide. Gross revenues in 1993 were expected to reach $56 million.

HealthPlus represented a multitude of services for employers. Although most members were in the HMO, it also included a PPO, indemnity, select provider network (SPN), administrative services and host of features tailor-made for individual employers.

The panel of physicians for HealthPlus were largely the same group of doctors who were in the Presbyterian Network. There was a limited number of non-Network physicians, and the plan was to phase these doctors out, thus eventually making the HealthPlus provider panel the same as the Network. This move towards provider panel symmetry is driven by the need to achieve efficiency in managing a panel (i.e., avoid duplication of efforts in provider relations, contracting, credentialing and recredentialing activities).

HealthPlus costs on a per member, per month basis have been stable since 1987. Costs have ranged from $73 in 1987 to $75 in 1992. Hospital admission rates for HealthPlus subscribers have dropped from 101 per 1,000 in 1987 to 67 per 1,000 in 1992. In terms of patient days, the HMO reported approximately 240 days per 1,000 members.

HealthPlus was profitable in 1989 through 1993. In 1992, there was $2.2 million in risk withholds for physicians and a surplus of $700,000; much of this also went to physicians. HealthPlus attributes its success to being responsive to customer demand and primary care physicians' management of health care resources in a cost-effective manner. The latter has been achieved primarily through bimonthly meetings of primary care physicians who meet in peer groups (Primary Provider Groups) to discuss costs, quality outcomes and medical policy.

Other Aspects of Presbyterian Healthcare Services

Continuous quality improvement. As noted above, physicians must agree to participate in CQI projects as a condition of membership in the Network. PHS and the Network place a high priority on CQI, a process that has been going on at PHS for over four years.

According to David Hildebrand, Clinical Project Coordinator, Quality Support Services, "PHS really incorporated the CQI philosophy as a business strategy when some of the employers in the area made inquiries into the system's involvement with quality improvement. This got our attention."

Hildebrand said that PHS has had nine teams that have completed CQI projects, and that 35 teams were in progress. He added, "Another six self destructed. We think there are probably another 50 teams functioning informally."

Hildebrand noted that PHS and the Network were looking at five or six clinical areas; all of these efforts involved Network physicians.

Information systems and database management. PHS and the Network were in the first few months of a five-year plan to develop a Network information system. Research and design to date has concentrated on the interviewing of over 40 individuals representing various perspectives of what the new system needs to provide. Marvin Feit, Chief Information Officer, calls the information system the nervous system of the Network.

The information system will focus on the patient and will include medical records, directories of providers and services, patient financial information, measures of quality, outcomes measurement, scheduling, clinical and medical practice support, billing and claims and marketing. It will bring together inpatient and outpatient care (e.g., a single patient record accessible at all Network locations).

One of the challenges facing the developers of the information system is to develop common definitions and patient identifiers (after considerable discussion, Social Security numbers will be used as the universal patient identification number). Other challenges include providing initial access through a common screen, security (making sure only individuals with a "need to know" can access information on a selective basis), and standardized computer equipment.

As a part of the system, Presbyterian's three hospitals will be linked with a fiber optic network. A new communications system linking physicians' offices with each other and with the hospitals also will be developed.

Resources required to develop the information system include 25 full-time equivalent staff members between 1993 and 1998 and capital expenditures of $5.7 million in 1994 and averaging $3 million annually in subsequent years.

Richard Barr summarized the need for a totally new approach to providing information. "It is essential that we function as a seamless organization. To do this we have to share clinical and financial data on a timely basis. We look upon the development of our new information system as a multi-year capital investment. The new system has to cover both inpatient and ambulatory care to be consistent with the way we are operating and intend to function in the future."

Major Accomplishments

In identifying Presbyterian's major successes to date, Dr. Koster identified the following:

- Family health care centers. "We have built a primary care base with facilities throughout the Albuquerque area. This definitely helps us market HealthPlus."

- Initial selection process completed. "We narrowed the panel from 600 to 400 physicians, and did it in a logical, systematic way."

- Market success measured in terms of HMO growth, direct contracting and serving as exclusive providers.

- Physician involvement high.

- Physician Management Board clearly creating integration.

- Cultures and organization in process of integration.

In addition to the successes identified by Dr. Koster, Dr. Horvath observed that physician members of the Network Board consistently take a broad perspective rather than focusing on their self interests. "It is amazing but it is happening." He said that there have been tremendous strides in the education of Network Board members in the role of governance. Also, members of the board were working well together.

From the perspective of physician participants in the Network, Dr. Horvath noted that there is strong support for physician involvement in Network management. He cited the increased number of physicians serving as program medical directors, and the fact that this is viewed as the beginning of integrating physicians into PHS operations.

Lessons Learned

Dr. Koster emphasized that the administrative expenses (start-up costs) involved with integration are significant; however, he said that PHS is looking at the long-term payoff. "The other alternative is to do nothing, and this is not an acceptable alternative."

Insights. Dr. Horvath cited the following:

- The Network is a <u>huge</u> undertaking. He noted that this effort is extremely labor intensive and requires major amounts of staff support.

- "The Network evolved as a response to what was happening in our market. Health care reform has fueled our progress."

- There are very complex issues in combining physician/hospital management cultures. "If we fail, this will be the primary reason."

- Physician involvement/commitment is crucial.

- The effort must be focused on the needs and expectations of the ultimate customers. "Payors and patients are the customers, and we have to stay focused on their needs."

- Evolution vs. revolution. "It seems like a revolution although we have been working on this since 1988."

- All must understand why integration creates advantages and work toward those goals. "It costs a lot of money to do this and we have to be able to talk about the payoff."

- Education and communication is overwhelmingly important with both physicians and administrators.

Obstacles. According to Dr. Koster, the major obstacles faced in the past and continuing to challenge PHS are:

- Rapidly changing schizophrenic legal environment. "Given the uncertainties of the legal environment, we have taken a conservative approach. Also, we are counting on our motivation of trying to do what is best for our customers to keep us out of trouble."

- "How to look and act integrated to customers when we are not all the way there yet."

- Selection of physicians for projects and contracting opportunities. Dr. Koster said this is still very contentious.

- Merger mentality/culture clash. "There tends to be a mentality after a merger that one group came and saved the other from disaster. This can be disruptive."

- Assimilating physician administrators.

- Traditional hospital manager fallout.

Issues for the Future

Dr. Horvath posed this question: "Is our strategy valid for the future?" His response was:

- Health care reform must occur at the delivery level.

- Organized care/premium mindset. This represents a major change for physicians and hospitals, and health care reform should promote this approach through capitation.

- Commitment to the community.

Conclusions

Dr. Koster discussed the "fear factor." He said it started in 1988 with primary care physicians who experienced the loss of patients to Lovelace. They also experienced added expenses in operating their medical practices and declining net incomes. However, he said, "The specialists still didn't get it." Dr. Koster referred to the health care "food chain" which begins with the primary care physician and ends with the specialist/hospital. He noted that since 1988 Presbyterian and the Network have made substantial progress in convincing specialists that they were losing their primary care base, and that this was a critically important problem.

Dr. Koster noted that the way PHS operates today is like driving a car with one foot on the gas pedal and the other on the brake. "The gas pedal is fee-for-service medicine where the more you pour it on, the more you make. The brake is capitation where the incentives <u>are to do less</u>. We are trying to do both at the same time, and it is frustrating."

Richard Barr, PHS President, concluded by saying, "Creating and managing the Network has been a huge undertaking. It is all consuming. We are creating a new organizational culture with physicians providing much of the leadership."

*Much of the information used to develop this case study was obtained from a briefing session presented by several PHS managers and physicians in Albuquerque on February 25, 1993. Additional information was provided by Kim Hedrick, Vice President, Network Development, and her staff; we appreciate their efforts.

Case Study #2

FARGO CLINIC/ST. LUKE'S HOSPITAL (MERITCARE)
Fargo, North Dakota

— Persons Interviewed —

Lloyd Smith, President and Chief Executive Officer, St. Luke's Hospital
John Paulsen, Executive Administrator, Fargo Clinic
Thomas Ahlin, MD, member of the Board of Directors, Fargo Clinic
Roger Gilbertson, MD, President, St. Luke's Association
Ruth Hanson, RN, Project Coordinator, RWJ Foundation Grant
Lawrence McGuire, Vice President, Human Resources, St. Luke's Hospital
Ronald Miller, MD, member of the Board of Directors, Fargo Clinic
Robert Montgomery, MD, Medical Director, Fargo Clinic and
    Chief of Staff, St. Luke's Hospital
Evelyn Quigley, Vice President, Patient Care Administration,
    St. Luke's Hospital
Wallace Radtke, MD, President and Chair of the Physician
    Service Corporation, the successor to the clinic
Carl Wall, Chairperson, St. Luke's Hospital, Board of Trustees

April, 1993

EXHIBIT A.

Location of St. Luke's Hospital and Fargo Clinic's Regional Centers

FARGO CLINIC/ST. LUKE'S HOSPITAL (MERITCARE)
Fargo, North Dakota*

In early 1993 the Fargo Clinic and St. Luke's Hospital were in the final stages of a merger. The restructured nonprofit association had been functioning since January 1, 1993 although the new organization would not officially be in place until July 1, 1993. (The post-merger organizations would be referred to as MeritCare Medical Group and MeritCare Hospital.) This case study focuses on the merger, including a description of the two entities prior to the merger, the reasons for the merger, the problems encountered during the merger process, and the benefits, both present and anticipated.

In introducing us to the merger, Lloyd Smith, CEO and President of St. Luke's Hospital, explained, "Although the hospital and clinic have been separate entities, we have been operating under the trade name of MeritCare since 1986. This merger positions our two organizations for the future. We can eliminate duplication of facilities and services, seek efficiencies in our operations, and present an integrated, cost-effective system of care that should be very appealing to payors."

John Q. Paulsen, Executive Administrator of the Fargo Clinic for the past 14 years, added, "We had a neighbor (the clinic and hospital are physically attached) and we decided we also wanted a financial partner. We think this is in the best interests of the community and our physicians."

Fargo Clinic and St. Luke's Hospital have been operating as separate but interrelated organizations since their foundings in the early part of this century. St. Luke's was a community not-for-profit hospital, and the Fargo Clinic was two for-profit corporations.

The Fargo-Moorhead Health Care Marketplace

The health care market served by Fargo-Moorhead physicians and hospitals includes a large portion of western Minnesota and eastern North Dakota. The location of St. Luke's Hospital and Fargo Clinic's regional centers is shown in Exhibit A.

Population and demographics. The Fargo-Moorhead Metropolitan Area straddles the Red River dividing North Dakota and Minnesota. The metropolitan area reported a 1990 population of approximately 153,000. The proportion of the population over the age of 65 was 10.5 percent (1990 Census data).

The total market area served by the Fargo Clinic and St. Luke's Hospital contained 368,000 persons. The proportion of the residents 65 years of age and older in the total market area was 14.6 percent; this was slightly above the national average (1990 Census).

Health plan coverage patterns. In early 1993, the marketplace served by the Fargo Clinic and St. Luke's Hospital was dominated by Medicare, Blue Cross and Blue Shield and traditional forms of health insurance coverage.

According to one person interviewed, the Fargo-Moorhead area is an "island of traditional health insurance coverage in the midst of a sea of managed care." Health maintenance organizations (HMOs) and preferred provider organizations (PPOs) represented less than five percent of the market. However, because of Fargo-Moorhead's proximity to the Minneapolis-St. Paul area, 250 miles to the east, health care providers and employers were well aware of the workings of HMOs and other forms of managed care.

Because of the older average age of the population in the market area, Medicare is proportionately more important, accounting for half of the inpatient admissions at St. Luke's Hospital and a substantial portion of the patients of physicians in the community.

Competition. The major competitors of the Fargo Clinic and St. Luke's Hospital are the Dakota Medical Center in Fargo, which includes both a hospital and multispecialty clinic, and the Heartland Medical Center (formerly St. John's Hospital), also in Fargo.

- *Dakota Medical Center.* In early 1993, the Dakota Hospital operated as a 194-bed facility offering a variety of services. The Dakota Clinic, Ltd. was the primary competitor of the Fargo Clinic, with 140 physicians on its staff. Dakota Clinic operated in over 25 locations in the Fargo-Moorhead area and in the surrounding two-state market area (e. g., Detroit Lakes and Moorhead, Minnesota and Wahpeton and Jamestown, North Dakota).

The Dakota Hospital had 25 percent of the inpatient admissions of Fargo-Moorhead hospitals in the July-September, 1992 quarter (latest data available). The occupancy rate of this hospital averaged between 55 and 60 percent in 1992.

• *Heartland Medical Center.* Heartland was the successor of St. John's Hospital in Fargo. St. John's Hospital and St. Ansgar Hospital in Moorhead were both part of the EcuNet system. However, St. Ansgar Hospital closed in 1992, and the ownership of the surviving organization (St. John's) changed to the Santa Fe Health Care Corporation. Heartland averaged 15 percent of admissions of the three Fargo-Moorhead hospitals (latest data available).

In addition, there were 12 small hospitals in the market area, as well as a limited number of private practice physicians. However, John Paulsen estimated that the Fargo Clinic included about 70 percent of the physicians in the outlying areas with many of the remaining doctors part of the Dakota Clinic.

Outreach activities. St. Luke's established three clinical networks and more were under development in early 1993. The networks included oncology (20 locations in the market area), emergency heart services (30 locations) and maternal child care (18 locations). According to Lloyd Smith, "This has had a favorable impact on the relationship between smaller community hospitals and St. Luke's, and has generated referrals. The Fargo Clinic physicians support these efforts."

Fargo Clinic

In 1993, the Fargo Clinic, one of the 11 largest multispecialty clinics in the country, had approximately 250 physicians in 30 locations, five in Fargo-Moorhead and 25 in smaller communities in North Dakota and Minnesota. Exhibit B shows the location of Fargo Clinic regional centers and satellite clinics serving North Dakota and Minnesota.

When asked why there were so many large clinics in the Upper Midwest, John Paulsen explained, "Over a long number of years, many of our physicians have taken their training at the Mayo Clinic in Rochester, where they have had an opportunity for exposure, firsthand, to the advantages of a group practice setting. Both physicians and patients like it."

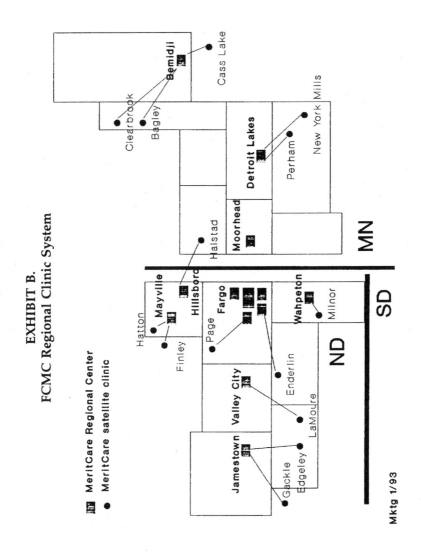

EXHIBIT B.
FCMC Regional Clinic System

EXHIBIT C.
Fargo Clinic Patient Visits, 1984-1992

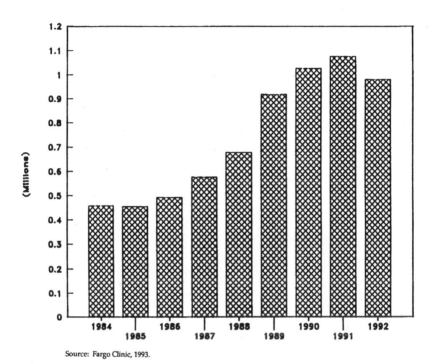

Source: Fargo Clinic, 1993.

EXHIBIT D.
Fargo Clinic Revenue, 1981-1992

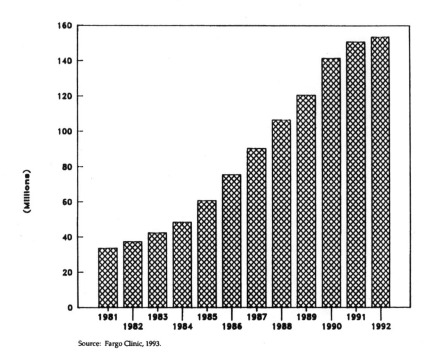

Source: Fargo Clinic, 1993.

Indicators of growth and size. The Fargo Clinic recorded over one million patient visits in 1992 (see trend in Exhibit C). Over half of the patients came from Minnesota.

Total clinic revenues were $150 million in 1992. This compared with $95 million five years earlier (see Exhibit D). The clinic had 1,700 employees in early 1993, up from 800 in 1980.

One of the physicians interviewed estimated that 70 percent of the physicians in the market area (outside of the Fargo-Moorhead area) were associated with the Fargo Clinic, with most of the remaining physicians on the staff of the Dakota Clinic in Fargo. This physician went on to estimate that within Fargo-Moorhead 85 to 90 percent of all physicians were in one of the large group practices (either Fargo Clinic or Dakota Clinic).

The clinic was actually made up of two corporations, Fargo Clinic Ltd. and Fargo Clinic Inc. The "Ltd" corporation is the medical practice which has over 200 shareholders, each with a single share. The "Inc" corporation owns and leases assets (buildings, equipment) and operates pharmacies. This corporation's stock is owned by a smaller number of physicians (and by Paulsen) in varying amounts depending on the desire of physicians to own stock in this entity. No new shares in "Inc." have been issued since 1988; therefore, most of the stock was owned by physicians who had been with the clinic for a number of years.

The mid-1980s expansion. Much of the growth of the Fargo Clinic occurred in 1983 through 1988, when several primary care practices became a part of the Fargo Clinic. John Paulsen noted, "The Fargo Clinic has traditionally not sought group practices for mergers. Normally, we have been approached by physicians who have an interest in joining the clinic. In 1983 there was a flurry of activity as the Dakota Clinic sought out small groups in smaller communities around Fargo-Moorhead. If we hadn't been willing to work with these groups, we probably would have been left at the starting gate. They now form a critical part of our system, especially its primary care component. And, they provide us with excellent geographic coverage of the region."

According to Paulsen, the issues raised by the primary care physicians joining the clinic included autonomy, value and payment for assets, income security and coping with bureaucracy (the clinic and its management). He added, "When the new primary care practices joined us, they became part of us legally and organizationally, even though the development of an integrated common culture took much longer to establish. However, this has changed. I would say today they are very much a part of the clinic." He went on to say that Wallace Radtke, MD, worked closely with these groups over a long period of time getting them involved with the Fargo Clinic. "Three out of eight members of the Fargo Clinic Ltd. board are from these primary care groups."

Dr. Radtke commented, "We recognized the need to expand our service area, and this is why we purchased these primary care practices. From the beginning we took the approach that these physicians were every bit as valuable as others on the clinic staff. We gave them the same voting rights, and they have been involved, from the beginning, in every aspect of the clinic."

The acquisition of the multispecialty Bemidji Clinic in 1988 was carried out for a different purpose. (Bemidji is 130 miles north east of Fargo.) John Paulsen explained that the Fargo Clinic's plan was to establish a core primary and secondary group in a larger community in Minnesota and to build a primary care referral base around it.

Admitting patients to hospitals. The decision of where a patient is to be hospitalized is always left up to individual Fargo Clinic physicians. For example, Fargo Clinic physicians in Mayville, North Dakota use their local hospital. Paulsen said, "They and their patients want to use it and support it. We encourage them to admit their patients wherever they want."

St. Luke's Hospital

St. Luke's Hospital operated 357 staffed beds, including 40 nursery bassinets, in early 1993. St. Luke's is a tertiary care facility and is the largest hospital in North Dakota. With 2,400 employees, it is also the largest private employer in the state. Over 99 percent of the admissions to St. Luke's Hospital are from physicians in the Fargo Clinic.

The hospital provided 103,177 days of inpatient care in fiscal year 1992 ending June 30. This was up slightly from fiscal year 1991. Emergency room visits exceeded 30,000 annually. The hospital recorded over 1,500 live births during the most recent 12-month period. An estimated 60 percent of the patients in the hospital were from Minnesota. In late 1992 the hospital had 60 percent of the inpatient admissions of the three hospitals in the Fargo-Moorhead area; this compared with 48 percent in 1987. Exhibit E shows the trend in market share (inpatient admissions) for St. Luke's Hospital, 1986 through the last quarter of 1992 (same as second quarter of the fiscal year).

Total revenues in fiscal year 1992 were $158 million, up from $86 million five years earlier. In its last fiscal year the hospital generated a surplus of $5.4 million. The hospital was in a solid financial position with assets of $115 million as of February 28, 1993, liabilities of $46 million and a fund balance of $69 million. Its debt service coverage ratio was 5.5, compared to an industry average of 3.7 times.

In addition to the acute care hospital, St. Luke's (and the clinic) operates the Roger Maris Cancer Center, a comprehensive outpatient facility providing treatment for cancer patients from a large area encompassing eastern North Dakota, western Minnesota and northern South Dakota.

History of Fargo Clinic/St. Luke's Hospital

Early history. St. Luke's Hospital, which was initially called the Lutheran Hospital Association, was established in May, 1905. The first hospital, named St. Luke's Hospital, had 35 beds and was opened in February, 1908. Three days after it opened the new hospital was filled to capacity. (This and subsequent historical information is from "Our History, 1905-Present," St. Luke's Association, MeritCare.)

The idea for what was to become the Fargo Clinic was presented to the board of trustees of St. Luke's Hospital on April 7, 1919 by Drs. Olaf Sand, Nils Tronnes, and other physicians. One of the first acts of the board was to find ways "to unite the two buildings with a tunnel and provide heat and other services to the Clinic."

From the beginning, the Fargo Clinic was located in buildings adjacent to St. Luke's Hospital. This has been a key factor in the close relationship of the two organizations over the past seven decades.

The 1980s — an era of joint ventures. Lloyd Smith joined St. Luke's Hospital in 1983, about the time of the introduction of Medicare's Prospective Payment System (DRGs). This was also the beginning of a period of extensive use of joint ventures by acute care hospitals and physicians across the country; the situation in Fargo was no different. "During my early years here I and others spent an awful lot of time putting together several joint ventures with the Fargo Clinic. These

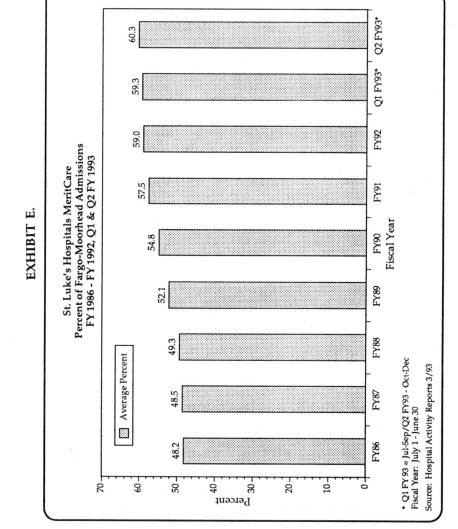

EXHIBIT E.

St. Luke's Hospitals MeritCare
Percent of Fargo-Moorhead Admissions
FY 1986 - FY 1992, Q1 & Q2 FY 1993

* Q1 FY 93 = Jul-Sep/Q2 FY93 - Oct-Dec
Fiscal Year: July 1 - June 30
Source: Hospital Activity Reports 3/93

included an outpatient surgery center, a home health service, a durable equipment company that sells and leases equipment over a three-state area, a child care center, magnetic resonance imaging service, and a property development company. All of these ventures have been financially successful."

The latest joint venture involved the creation of the Roger Maris Cancer Center. Smith said, "This venture was unbelievably complicated. As with our other ventures, the cancer center has been very successful. We are seeing 100 new patients a month."

The name change. In 1986, after considerable discussion, the Fargo Clinic and St. Luke's Hospital agreed to adopt the name "MeritCare." Lloyd Smith referred to this as a new "family name." It was developed primarily for marketing and corporate identification purposes.

According to John Paulsen, the Fargo Clinic has found the MeritCare name especially valuable in smaller communities. "Given the concern of people living in small towns about being taken over or dominated by Fargo, it was not desirable to refer to our clinics in these smaller communities as branches of the Fargo Clinic. The name MeritCare worked much better for us, and we have incorporated it into all of our advertising and corporate identification materials. We are very pleased with what it has accomplished."

Paulsen added, "Going to the MeritCare name really started the process of the two organizations thinking of themselves as a single entity."

Ron Miller, MD, and member of the board of the Fargo Clinic, said, "When I first heard the name MeritCare, I wasn't all that impressed. But, it has really caught on and is definitely an asset. Before we were referred to as 'St. Luke's doctors.'"

The 1989 merger discussions. Lloyd Smith said that the factors triggering the merger were:

- Health care reform.

- Changes in the marketplace.

- Declining reimbursement for both physicians and the hospital (half of the patients in St. Luke's Hospital are covered by Medicare).

- Difficulty in structuring and managing joint ventures. "The Federal government has been making it more difficult to go down the road we had chosen."

- A desire to more effectively and efficiently serve our patients.

Carl Wall, Chairperson of the St. Luke's Hospital board of trustees, described the reasons for the merger in different terms. "First, there was the strong possibility of health care reform. Second, we were experiencing declining reimbursement for both physicians and the hospital." He went on, "If we are on the same page — the clinic and hospital — it will lead to higher quality of care and a slower rise in costs for the community. This is in the public interest."

John Paulsen observed that at about this same time he and Dr. Radtke were meeting with their counterparts in the Clinic Club (an informal group of 11 large clinics in the US that meets annually). "It was at one of these meetings that we first began to discuss ideas relating to potential mergers between group practices and hospitals."

Dr. Radtke noted that the clinic board evaluated the possibility of going it alone, but this seemed illogical. "We had the horizontal (geographic) integration but we needed to be vertically integrated."

One of the initial acts in the 1989 merger discussions was to hire Booz Allen & Hamilton to assist in the effort. This firm provided a series of reports recommending that the two entities proceed with the merger. According to Lloyd Smith, the primary reasons cited were strategic, and that reducing expenses should not be the primary motivation.

During the period when merger discussions were taking place, the management and board representatives of the two organizations traveled to Seattle to review how the Virginia Mason merger had been accomplished, to San Diego to visit with representatives of Sharp Rees-Stealy, and to Minneapolis-St. Paul for visits with the Ramsey Clinic.

Despite the initial efforts and interest in merger, the discussions bogged down and ceased altogether in late 1990. Lloyd Smith said, "No one was angry. We just were not making much progress and the people involved were beginning to wonder whether or not the time was right for a merger. There was also concern and uncertainty with such organizations when comparing the differences, cultures, and governance styles. It was nothing unusual, just the traditional set of relationships you find in most places."

From the Fargo Clinic perspective, John Paulsen said, "After the discussions went on for about two years they began to deteriorate. We had problems determining how to bring together two such different entities." He went on to say, "The doctors owned the clinic and were solely responsible for its destiny. Some physicians were not sure they wanted to give up even some control of their own destinies. These were emotional issues."

Paulsen added, "When the discussions ended, there was great regret that they had failed. During the 18-month hiatus some physicians softened their positions on some of the issues. Additionally, the health care environment was changing rapidly."

He also noted that after negotiations had ceased, some of the Fargo Clinic physicians were asking themselves, "Are we losing a window of opportunity? As a result, we came back to the table better prepared to negotiate."

The recent merger negotiations. In June, 1991, just six months after negotiations had ended, one of the hospital board members raised the merger issue again at a board retreat. After discussion, it was agreed that the hospital would try to pick up the negotiations in early 1992.

Dr. Miller said that from his perspective there were three reasons for moving ahead with the merger: "First, it would provide the greatest long-term viability for both the hospital and clinic. Secondly, it would enhance the long-term income prospects for the clinic staff. And third, it should strengthen our role in health care delivery in the area. I feel that physicians will be better off both in terms of income and flexibility of practice style."

When negotiations resumed, both the clinic and hospital were represented by five individuals. However, Lloyd Smith said this did not work as well as had been hoped and progress was slow. "Also, we favored a structured approach, but the clinic was not accustomed to this. They felt pressured. Things worked better when the agenda and assignments were more informal."

Both the clinic and hospital employed legal counsel to advise them on how to accomplish the merger and avoid problems with private inurement, antitrust and safe harbor legislation. Lloyd Smith said, "In the early stages of negotiations, the law firms tended to view their roles as representing the entities paying their bills. However, when it became obvious that the merger would occur, they tended to view their client as the new merged association."

Lloyd Smith added, "I can't overemphasize the complexities of this merger. Even though we had the best legal counsel possible, every time we opened a door we would find three more that were closed. And, we didn't even know they were there! Then, we had to find the right combinations for these doors."

As progress in the negotiations slowed, responsibility was delegated to four individuals — Lloyd Smith and Bruce Briggs (who was in charge of planning and related activities) representing St. Luke's Hospital and John Paulsen and Dr. Radtke representing Fargo Clinic. Lloyd Smith said, "This was a key turning point. It was much easier to get to know each other, build trust, and attack the key issues."

John Paulsen agreed. "The smaller group worked much better. We could become more intimate; there was less posturing. There was a frankness and candor that helped us get through some difficult problems."

Paulsen noted that Dr. Radtke made a major effort to keep all physicians well informed of progress and decisions. "We had monthly letters to all physicians from Dr. Radtke, and weekly briefings with our board. We also had monthly dinner meetings with about 60 department chairpersons and heads of the regional clinics to keep them up to date on the status of the negotiations."

Paulsen identified six critical issues from a physician perspective that came up during the negotiations:

- Price
- Governance (control)
- Management structure
- Autonomy
- Income/salaries
- Pension plan

On the latter point, Lloyd Smith said, "The pension plan was almost a deal breaker. The clinic had a more generous plan, and it had performed substantially better than the hospital's plan. The ERISA and other legal requirements made retaining the group practice pension plan a very complex situation. In the end we agreed to develop a common plan for both institutions."

Financial Implications

The shareholders of Fargo Clinic, Ltd. (the medical practice) and Fargo Clinic Inc. (the owner of buildings, equipment and other assets) will receive cash and notes payable for their shares.

As noted earlier, around 200 physicians each own one share of Fargo Clinic Ltd., and each will receive $50,000, the same amount they paid in when they became shareholders. The payment will be $25,000 at the time of the merger with the remainder payable over two years.

Shareholders of Fargo Clinic Inc. will receive notes payable from the St. Luke's Association based on the book value of the stock owned. These notes are payable over 10 years. John Paulsen said, "The appraisals carried out to establish the value of these assets determined that the ultimate price agreed upon could be well supported."

Mission of the St. Luke's Association

As of early 1993 the restructured association was operating but had not yet adopted a formal mission statement. According to Roger Gilbertson, MD, newly-elected President of the Saint Luke's Association, this will be one of the first tasks. He summarized the mission of the new organization as, "Functioning as the premier integrated health care system in our market area."

Evelyn Quigley, Vice President, Patient Care Administration for St. Luke's Hospital, said that it is important for the Association to develop a joint mission statement. "We have different perspectives about our missions and what we are trying to accomplish. This is understandable. But, now we have a chance to come together and this is exciting."

In its April 1989 assessment of the potential for the two organizations to merge, Booz•Allen & Hamilton Inc. suggested the following as the shared visions of the Fargo Clinic and St. Luke's Hospital:

• Continue to develop as an integrated provider of a full range of high quality medical services, encompassing primary through tertiary care, in selected geographic markets.

- Continue to develop as the premier tertiary care center serving western Minnesota, central and eastern North Dakota, and northeast South Dakota.

- Provide a challenging, rewarding environment that will motivate the highest quality health care professionals and managers to be part of the MeritCare network of services.

Governance

Organization and governance before merger. The organization chart for the Fargo Clinic is shown as Exhibit F.

Regarding the hospital organizational structure, Larry McGuire, Vice President for Human Resources, said that the hospital reorganized in 1992 and eliminated two layers of management. One of the jobs eliminated was that of chief operating officer. "Today we are much more decentralized."

Organization and governance in early 1993. Exhibit G is the organizational chart for the St. Luke's Association and the two surviving hospital and clinic boards. Dr. Gilbertson is President of the Association with Lloyd Smith serving as Executive Vice President. Gilbertson began his new duties January 1, 1993. His medical practice is expected to take one quarter of his time with the new job requiring three quarters.

Lloyd Smith continues to serve as President, CEO and Chair of the hospital and board, now reconstituted as primarily a management board with nine hospital executive staff members, clinic president, association president, the Executive Administrator of the Fargo Clinic (John Paulsen), and two community representatives.

The clinic board, includes eight physicians from the clinic, Association President (Dr. Gilbertson), hospital President (Smith), another member of the hospital executive management team, and two community members. The President and Chair of this board is Dr. Radtke.

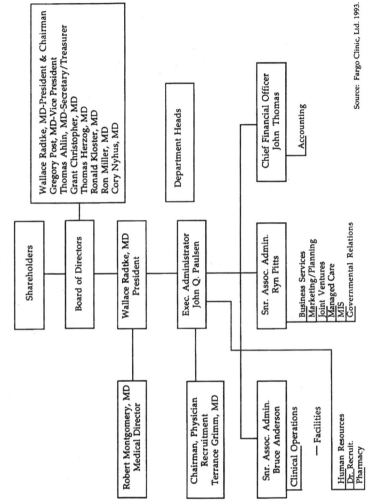

EXHIBIT F.
Structure of Fargo Clinic, Ltd.

Shareholders

Board of Directors

Wallace Radtke, MD-President & Chairman
Gregory Post, MD-Vice President
Thomas Ahlin, MD-Secretary/Treasurer
Grant Christopher, MD
Thomas Herzog, MD
Ronald Kloster, MD
Ron Miller, MD
Cory Nyhus, MD

Wallace Radtke, MD
President

Robert Montgomery, MD
Medical Director

Exec. Administrator
John Q. Paulsen

Chairman, Physician
Recruitment
Terrance Grimm, MD

Department Heads

Snr. Assoc. Admin.
Ryn Pitts

Business Services
Marketing/Planning
Joint Ventures
Managed Care
MIS
Governmental Relations

Snr. Assoc. Admin.
Bruce Anderson

Clinical Operations
— Facilities

Human Resources
Dr. Recruit.
Pharmacy

Chief Financial Officer
John Thomas

Accounting

Source: Fargo Clinic, Ltd. 1993.

EXHIBIT G.
St. Luke's Association Organizational Chart

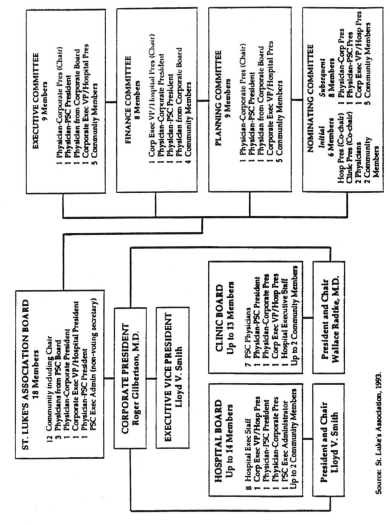

EXECUTIVE COMMITTEE
9 Members

1 Physician-Corporate Pres (Chair)
1 Physician-PSC President
1 Physician from Corporate Board
1 Corporate Exec VP/Hospital Pres
5 Community Members

FINANCE COMMITTEE
8 Members

1 Corp Exec VP/Hospital Pres (Chair)
1 Physician-Corporate President
1 Physician-PSC President
1 Physician from Corporate Board
4 Community Members

PLANNING COMMITTEE
9 Members

1 Physician-Corporate Pres (Chair)
1 Physician-PSC President
1 Physician from Corporate Board
1 Corporate Exec VP/Hospital Pres
5 Community Members

NOMINATING COMMITTEE

Initial
6 Members

Hosp Pres (Co-chair)
Clinic Pres (Co-chair)
2 Physicians
2 Community Members

Subsequent
8 Members

1 Physician-Corp Pres
1 Physician-PSC Pres
1 Corp Exec VP/Hosp Pres
5 Community Members

ST. LUKE'S ASSOCIATION BOARD
18 Members

12 Community including Chair
3 Physicians from PSC Board
1 Physician-Corporate President
1 Corporate Exec VP/Hospital President
1 Physician-PSC President
PSC Exec Admin (non-voting secretary)

CORPORATE PRESIDENT
Roger Gilbertson, M.D.

EXECUTIVE VICE PRESIDENT
Lloyd V. Smith

HOSPITAL BOARD
Up to 14 Members

8 Hospital Exec Staff
1 Corp Exec VP/Hosp Pres
1 Physician-PSC President
1 Physician-Corporate Pres
1 PSC Exec Administrator
Up to 2 Community Members

President and Chair
Lloyd V. Smith

CLINIC BOARD
Up to 13 Members

7 PSC Physicians
1 Physician-PSC President
1 Physician-Corporate Pres
1 Corp Exec VP/Hosp Pres
1 Hospital Executive Staff
Up to 2 Community Members

President and Chair
Wallace Radtke, M.D.

Source: St. Luke's Association, 1993.

Lloyd Smith said, "Under this new structure we have substantial crossover between the hospital and clinic. For example, I am now on the clinic board; before the merger the hospital was not represented on the clinic's board of directors. Also, the hospital board includes the clinic president plus John Paulsen."

Administrative Coordinating Council. Smith characterized this as a joint senior management group that has been meeting for four months. This group is responsible for resolving disputes and assigning responsibilities between the clinic and hospital. As of early 1993, the Council had identified 20 areas for consolidation.

Factors Influencing the Number and Mix of Physicians

In looking back, John Paulsen said that the primary care practice acquisitions a decade ago represented one of the most profound periods of change during his 43 years with the Fargo Clinic. He noted that in 1982 the Fargo Clinic had no family practice physicians. "In 1992 we had 63 family doctors and they represented the largest specialty group on the staff. I think this is a step in the right direction and it positions us well for the future."

Dr. Radtke agreed with this assessment of the importance of building a primary care base. He said that he expects the proportion of primary care physicians in the clinic to continue to increase. "I can see primary care physicians representing 60 to 70 percent of our staff within a few years." In response to how this will affect medical specialists, he said, "It won't be a sudden, overnight change. We hope that the mix of specialties in the clinic will evolve naturally based on market demands."

At the time this case study was prepared, specialists at the Fargo Clinic were subsidizing primary care physicians. In other words, the revenues generated by primary care doctors were not sufficient to cover the overhead and compensation levels (usually in the $100,000 to $120,000 range). This was recognized and accepted as being necessary for the clinic to continue to function and serve the needs of the market area, and to generate referrals for specialists.

Dr. Miller said that the University of North Dakota medical school has been producing about 50 physicians per year and this has helped in recruiting new doctors to the area. He also said, "The Fargo Clinic has a pretty good mix of primary care physicians and specialists, although we are short on OB/GYN and one or two other specialties."

Lloyd Smith does not feel that the clinic has too many specialists or is out of balance. "I think the physician mix is about right for the health care environment at the present time."

Physician Compensation

Physician compensation levels at the Fargo Clinic are influenced by the recommendations of a committee of physicians to the board of the clinic. This process is unlikely to change under the merger.

Factors influencing physician compensation. The Fargo Clinic physician committee responsible for analyzing compensation patterns and making annual recommendations relies on a "market-driven approach." This means that committee members evaluate a variety of data sources, including the Medical Group Management Association (MGMA) productivity surveys, and data from other members of the Clinic Club, in arriving at reasonable levels of physician payment.

Dr. Miller said, "People who come here know they are not going to make as much as they might in another situation." Dr. Radtke agreed: "If someone is looking to make a big salary, they had better look elsewhere."

This is a key issue related to future physician compensation, when it is expected that primary care physicians may be rewarded more for their services, and specialist compensation may decrease. According to Dr. Miller, "With our system we should be able to make these adjustments with relative ease. We are not locked into a system that pays specialists more; the marketplace will be the key driver."

The compensation issue. As a part of the merger, St. Luke's Association agreed to support stabilizing physicians' compensation at current levels for the first three years. Due to regulatory constraints, this became a very complex and difficult issue. To arrive at such a methodology meant involving legal consultation throughout the process. However, the parties were successful at arriving at something that was felt to be a positive solution.

Range of physician compensation. John Paulsen and others indicated that the range of physician compensation at the Fargo Clinic is narrow compared with most multispecialty clinics. Up until 1988, the range was 100 to 150 percent. In other words, the compensation of specialists did not exceed that of primary care physicians by more than 50 percent. If a primary care physician earned $110,000 (the low end), specialists would not earn more than $165,000. Because of the need to pay more to attract certain specialists, these guidelines have been relaxed somewhat over the past four years. Dr. Radtke estimated that approximately 20 percent of the specialists on the clinic staff are above the upper range.

Combining Support Services

Even though the 1989 consultants' study predicted that economies of operation were available through the merger, the consulting firm indicated that these savings would be relatively small compared with other potential benefits (e.g., combined strategic planning, positioning for managed care contracting, ability to improve quality of care and measure outcomes).

John Paulsen said, "Overhead expenses in the future are a major concern to our physicians. We need to reduce duplication and cut costs. We have already identified several areas for consolidations." He cited the following:

- Radiology
- Information systems
- Plant operations
- Human resources
- Planning and marketing
- Housekeeping
- Utility management
- Maintenance of equipment
- Telecommunications

The hospital and clinic have had comparable compensation systems since 1980, and wages and salaries do not differ markedly. According to Larry McGuire, the big difference is in benefits, primarily the pension plan. Both organizations are self insured for health insurance with Blue Cross and Blue Shield of North Dakota providing administrative services. Job evaluation procedures and forms are comparable.

HMO Experience

The Fargo Clinic started MedCenters HMO in 1985. The HMO was managed by American MedCenters, an HMO management company based in Minneapolis.

Dr. Montgomery, who was on the board of the HMO at the time, said, "These people were really good at one thing — marketing. Within two or three years they had enrolled close to 40,000 subscribers." According to Dr. Montgomery, the problem with the HMO management company was the "lack of data systems, lack of training for physicians on how to function within an HMO environment, and the lack of deep pockets." He added, "We wanted to do it ourselves; we should have brought in the hospital as our partner."

When the decision was made in 1988 to close down the HMO, the clinic had invested close to $10 million into the venture. One of the Fargo Clinic physicians said, "In hind sight we should have brought in the hospital, and we should have kept going. Look where we would be today if we hadn't given up. But, the financial drain on physician incomes was just too much. It was a hard-learned lesson and I hope it will pay off for us in the future."

John Paulsen said that he anticipates a re-entry into managed care. "The fee-for-service environment is coming to an end, and we will be positioned to participate in risk contracting, either through owning our own financing mechanism, or in conjunction with other organizations."

Other Aspects of the Fargo Clinic/St. Luke's Hospital

Continuous quality improvement. Dr. Gilbertson said that the hospital is ahead of the clinic in terms of implementing CQI because it has an infrastructure carrying out quality improvement. "I think the clinic will come along fast; some of the people over there are interested and knowledgeable about CQI."

Speaking of the clinic, Dr. Miller noted, "We are well positioned for the future in most areas, but I am afraid we are lacking in CQI."

Outcomes measurement. With its Clinical/Financial Information System (C/FIS), the hospital was ahead of the clinic in terms of being able to assess outcomes and compare costs with benefits. (The C/FIS was originally developed by Voluntary Hospitals of America's North Central Region; St. Luke's Hospital is a part of this alliance.)

Dr. Miller added that the clinic has done little in outcomes measurement, and that "it needs to do more. We are going to be evaluated on this basis in the future, so we had better get ready."

Evelyn Quigley noted that in the future, "We need to focus on the health status of the people being served rather than on treating sick people. Health care reform will push us in that direction, and I personally believe it is the right way to go."

Patient-focused care. St. Luke's Hospital was one of 20 hospitals receiving a grant from the Robert Wood Johnson (RWJ) Foundation to develop and implement a five-year plan for restructuring hospital nursing services. According to Quigley, "Work supported by the grant has led to new thinking about the future of the hospital, the way care has been delivered, and the way it will be delivered in the future." She went on, "The hospital has more changing to do than the clinic. We have focused on high-tech treatment, but this may not be our future."

Ruth Hanson, RN and project coordinator for the RWJ Foundation grant, said that nurses are much happier with the new approach to delivering care. "It puts nurses out into the patient areas, and they feel closer to patients. They do less running around and more productive work."

In discussing patient-focused care and CQI, Robert Montgomery, MD (serving as both Medical Director of the Fargo Clinic and Chief of Staff for the hospital) said, "You have to avoid labels, and don't build up expectations by a lot of preselling. It is better to use a low key approach. Just invite physicians to a meeting where you are going to discuss ways to improve something in the hospital, and they are more likely to come, enjoy themselves and participate on an on-going basis."

Information Systems. Lloyd Smith said, "Information systems are the key to the future in health care, including our new organization. We have to be able to integrate the systems of the clinic and hospital. We are in the process of evaluating instituting a chief information officer position in order to help us get this mammoth task accomplished."

Dr. Gilbertson agreed that the information systems of the two organizations have to be integrated and upgraded, and "this will be expensive."

The Fargo Clinic and St. Luke's Hospital have both invested heavily in separate information systems. This means that to take advantage of the opportunities created by the merger, a new integrated information system involving patient data at both the clinic and hospital level must be designed and implemented. The required capital investment will be large -- several million dollars a year for several years.

Corporate Culture. Regarding the corporate culture of the hospital, Larry McGuire said the hospital has been empowering employees, encouraging more risk taking, working with self-managed groups, driving information to lower levels, and removing a sense of entitlement. On the latter point, he cited a bonus system that had been in effect for many years that was based on seniority. "We recently dropped it and put out the message that we were going to pay for productivity."

On another matter relating to corporate culture, Thomas Ahlin, MD, a member of the board of the Fargo Clinic, said, "The hospital board is largely made up of community people, and they are not directly involved with health care. They tend to view being a trustee the same as being on a corporate board. And, they are dependent on the hospital CEO to provide them with the information they need to make decisions. They usually go along with management's recommendations, and there is usually little controversy in the decision-making process. They don't like to ruffle each others feathers."

"In the case of the clinic board, we are all involved in health care, and the success of the organization represents our livelihood. We get a lot more feedback from our shareholders (the 200+ physicians who own stock in the clinic). When they have a complaint or suggestion they tend to be vocal. They don't always get their own way, but at least we give them a hearing. We accept this as the normal way of doing business as a director of a clinic."

He went on, "When I first thought about the affairs of the Fargo Clinic being influenced by a lay board, my reaction was negative. But, the more I thought about it, having a lay board in an influential position didn't bother me. Being physicians I thought we could influence the board's deliberations and decision making. I thought as long as we are doing a good job they will take us seriously."

Dr. Montgomery discussed the different cultures of the two organizations along these lines. "You have to remember that the clinic is a for-profit business and the clinic administrator works for more than 200 shareholders. The board of the clinic meets weekly and is very involved with operations. This leads to a certain management style." He went on, "In the case of the hospital, the CEO reports to the board of trustees, a group of community leaders who have no direct financial interest in the hospital. This group usually meets monthly and the agenda is presented by hospital management."

Benefits Expected from the Merger

Several of the individuals interviewed as part of this case study cited anticipated benefits of the merger. Larry McGuire, VP for Human Resources, cited five advantages of the new organization:

- Assurance of a base of physicians.

- Advantages of an integrated delivery system, including the ability to compete for managed care contracts.

- Efficiencies of operation, such as consolidation of departments.

- Streamlining of administration.

- Ability to throw more financial and human resources at issues and opportunities.

Dr. Gilbertson cited three primary payoffs from the merger: (1) integrated, cost-effective health care system, (2) establishment of a breadth and depth of services to handle the health care needs of a defined population (capitation), and (3) economies of scale.

Evelyn Quigley noted that one of the reasons that the merger makes sense is because the hospital has been focusing on its role as a tertiary care facility, and the clinic has been concentrating on primary care. "Between the two of us, we have the matter pretty well covered. But," she said, "it will take both perspectives to be successful in the future."

Quigley also talked about the difference in thinking between a hospital and medical group. "We are really happy when visits to the emergency room are up; this drives revenues. However, when we look behind the numbers, many of these patients shouldn't be using the emergency room; they should be treated in physician's offices. Under the new structure we can have a fruitful discussion about this problem."

Dr. Montgomery cited these benefits of the merger:

- "We — the clinic and hospital — won't be duplicating.

- We will have access to capital. As with most medical group practices, we have little ability to accumulate capital. By joining with the hospital, we partially solve this problem.

- Most customers already view the two as one organization.

- We will be able to conduct strategic planning together."

Lessons Learned

Proceeding with smaller negotiating teams. Lloyd Smith said there were several important lessons he learned from the process of negotiating with the clinic. The first was that it is better to proceed with a small group. Even though the second phase of the negotiations began with five representatives from each organization, he felt this was too many people and that progress was slow. Once it was agreed to delegate negotiations to four individuals the process began to click. "This is where we really made the breakthroughs on the difficult issues," Smith said.

Tackle leadership issues early. Another lesson learned, according to Smith, was that it is important to tackle the difficult issue of leadership of the new organization early. "If you don't put it on the table and discuss it right off, it is always in the background and it influences what people say and how they interact. It is best to confront the issue of leadership up front and get it resolved. Things move much more smoothly if you do it this way."

Dr. Radtke agreed. "The leadership issues that come up in a merger of this type are painful. My advice to anyone contemplating this sort of arrangement is to face the issues of who is going to fill what role right up front."

Sense of urgency. Carl Wall, Chairman of the St. Luke's board, said that one lesson learned was the lack of urgency in the merger negotiations. "I think we could and should have moved faster. Health care groups just starting down this road won't have the luxury of the extended time period we had to get the job done. The pressures are becoming great to move more faster." He also believes that an outside facilitator would have helped move the process ahead more quickly.

Flexibility. Wall also talked of the importance of keeping the agreements and relationships flexible. "We didn't want to get locked into any fixed agreement relative to what we could or could not do; we needed to stay loose and flexible, and maintain our ability to respond to changes and opportunities as they presented themselves."

Issues for the Future

In 1992, the State of Minnesota passed legislation affecting the delivery of health care in the state. This included the establishment of several integrated service networks (ISNs). ISNs are HMO-like plans that deliver a package of benefits at a predetermined price (capitation). Lloyd Smith said, "Since over half of our business comes from Minnesota, we have to position the hospital and clinic to compete for contracts from these ISNs."

At the time this case study was prepared, the Association had hired a consultant to assist in preparing the new organization for a future involving more managed care. Smith said, "We are definitely positioning ourselves to take on risk contracting. Will we start an HMO? It is not out of the question."

Dr. Radtke concluded by saying, "The only way for us to survive is to become streamlined and more cost effective. The merger placed us in a strengthened position to meet the demands of the marketplace. He pointed out that Minnesota hospitals and physicians are "moving into the Minnesota portion of our service area." He also said that the new merged organization should be more capable of responding to health care reform.

---

*Lloyd Smith, President and CEO of St. Luke's Hospital, and John Q. Paulsen, Executive Administrator, Fargo Clinic, provided much of the background and administrative support for this case study. We thank both of them, and their excellent support staffs, for their interest and cooperation.

Case Study #3

MARSHFIELD CLINIC/
ST. JOSEPH'S HOSPITAL
Marshfield, Wisconsin

— Persons Interviewed —

Richard Leer, MD, President, Marshfield Clinic
Fritz Wenzel, Advisor to the President, Marshfield Clinic
Peter Bauer, Director, Information Systems, Marshfield Clinic
Robert DeVita, Senior Associate Director, Marshfield Clinic
Reed Hall, General Counsel, Marshfield Clinic
William Maurer, MD, Medical Director, Greater Marshfield
      Community Health Plan
Ronald Pfannerstill, Director, Financial Affairs,
      Marshfield Clinic
Michael Schmidt, Executive Vice President and interim CEO,
      St. Joseph's Hospital
Frederic Wesbrook, MD, Medical Director, Marshfield Clinic

May, 1993

EXHIBIT A
Location of Marshfield Clinic

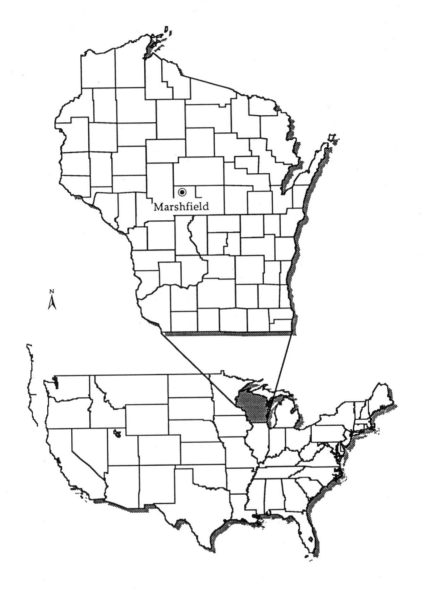

MARSHFIELD CLINIC/
ST. JOSEPH'S HOSPITAL
Marshfield, Wisconsin

The Marshfield Clinic, with 392 physicians, is one of the largest medical groups in the United States. It is in close proximity to St. Joseph's Hospital (525 beds). Physicians associated with the Marshfield Clinic account for more than 99 percent of the inpatient admissions to the hospital.

Marshfield, a community of 20,000, is located in central Wisconsin. Exhibit A shows the location of Marshfield in the state.

The Marshfield Health Care Marketplace

Description of the area served. There are an estimated 800,000 persons in the service area of the Marshfield Clinic. The average age of residents is above the national average; therefore, dependence on Medicare as a payment source is higher than normal.

Health plan coverage patterns. Most of the residents of the service area are covered by either Medicare or commercial insurance (usually traditional indemnity coverage). Managed care, primarily health maintenance organizations (HMOs), does not have the same degree of market penetration as in many other parts of the country; it was believed to be less than 10 percent.

The payor mix of St. Joseph's Hospital was indicative of the types of health plan coverage patterns in the region. In fiscal year 1992 (ending September 30), just over half of all patient days were accounted for by Medicare patients. Medicaid patients represented 9.5 percent of all patient days. Commercial insurance represented 24 percent of total patient days, and Blue Cross and Blue Shield accounted for just over four percent. Only 8.5 percent of the patients were enrolled in an HMO. (Exhibit D, presented later, shows changes in the hospital's payor mix over the past five years.)

Competing clinics and physicians. There are a large hospital and a medical group in Wausau, 30 miles northeast of Marshfield. The Wausau Hospital Center has 315 beds and advertises that its market area covers

12 counties.   There are 155 physicians on the medical staff of this hospital.

The Mayo Clinic recently purchased the Midelfort Clinic (60 physicians) and the Luther Hospital in Eau Claire, 70 miles west of Marshfield.   This is viewed (by physicians and administrators of the Marshfield Clinic) as an aggressive move.

The Gundersen Clinic (270 physicians) in La Crosse is 80 miles southwest of Marshfield and is not viewed as a prime competitor of either Marshfield Clinic or St. Joseph's Hospital. Its focus has been on southwest Wisconsin, Iowa and Minnesota.

There are large hospitals and clinics in Milwaukee (180 miles south east), in Madison (140 miles south) and in the Green Bay/Fox River Valley area (two hours drive to the east).   The Duluth Clinic (170 physicians) is developing a regional health care system that is also reaching into northern Wisconsin.

Shortage of primary care physicians in rural areas. There continues to be a shortage of primary care physicians in smaller communities in central and northern Wisconsin. It was estimated that there were 100 vacancies for primary care doctors in northern Wisconsin.

History of Marshfield Clinic

Founding of the Marshfield Clinic. The Marshfield Clinic was founded in 1916 by six physicians, all in general practice, who later became trained in various specialties of medicine and surgery. As stated by the founders, "The aim of the organization was to give better and more efficient service to the public and to do it in a scientific way in order to compete with the medical centers in the larger cities."

The founders also decided that although the clinic was initially a for-profit corporation, the assets would be held in trust, and that the sale of the assets could not inure to the benefits of the owners. They declared research and education in the service of medicine essential values of their new organization.

Early growth. The clinic grew slowly during the 1920s and 1930s. Several physicians were added to the staff, including Stephen Epstein, MD, an internationally-known dermatologist, who became the first president of the Marshfield Clinic Medical Research Foundation.

The advent of World War II slowed the growth of the clinic. However, in the 1950s growth resumed, fueled by the number of physicians who obtained their training through the GI Bill. An equal salary plan (all physicians earned the same amount), democratic governance system, and the research foundation were born during this period.

When Fritz Wenzel joined the clinic as a biochemist in 1953, there were 23 physicians. He became Executive Director of Marshfield Clinic in 1976. At that time, the organization had expanded to 160 physicians. There were just under 400 physicians when he moved from that position to that of Advisor to the President in 1993.

Change in location/new buildings. From 1926 through 1975, the clinic was housed in a building located on the main street of Marshfield. A 220,000 square foot facility was constructed next to St. Joseph's Hospital in 1975. With additional buildings added during the 1984 through 1989 period, the clinic expanded to 654,000 square feet in its main location and to 21 other sites outside the central facility.

Changes in legal structure. In 1980, the clinic was converted from a for-profit business corporation to a 501(c)4 corporation. This was an interim step. In 1987 the clinic applied for and received designation as a 501(c)3 corporation. Reed Hall, the Clinic's General Counsel, reported, "This was important because it meant we could bring the research and education foundation back into the clinic (it had been set up as a separate non-profit organization in 1959). We could also use the tax exempt bond market and this saves us $10 million a year in interest payments and tax savings."

Hall also said that the clinic is constantly on guard against fraud and abuse problems. "We make sure when we deal with the hospital that we pay fair market value for property or rentals. We try to live beyond reproach."

Marshfield Clinic in early 1993. An interview with Frederic Wesbrook, MD, Medical Director of the clinic, revealed that the clinic serves just under one million patients per year. "I believe this represents a base of around 200,000 people." Exhibit B shows several key volume indicators for the Marshfield Clinic, 1988 through 1992.

Exhibit B.
Key Indicators, Marshfield Clinic
1988-1992 (Year-ending September 30)

Indicator	1988	1989	1990	1991	1992
Total Revenue (millions)	$125.2	$144.0	$174.4	$206.3	$231.7
Expenses (millions)	118.5	135.8	166.6	199.9	224.1
Net Earnings (millions)	6.7	8.2	7.8	6.4	7.7
Patient Encounters (thousands)	630.1	676.9	783.0	879.5	966.5
Number of Physicians	261	319	328	378	393
Number of Employees	1,649	1,898	2,112	2,418	2,499

Source: Marshfield Clinic, April, 1993.

About one-third of the patients using the clinic in early 1993 came from a clinic-operated HMO. Another quarter had commercial insurance, and close to 20 percent were covered by Medicare. The remainder of the patients were Medicaid and fee-for-service.

The mission of Marshfield Clinic in 1993 was, "To serve patients through accessible, quality health care, research and education."

Governance. All physicians who have successfully completed two one-year contracts are invited to become shareholders, and each has one vote. The shareholders elect a president and a nine-person executive committee. The president can serve six one-year terms. Other members of the executive committee serve three-year terms.

The Marshfield Clinic Executive Committee functions as the board of directors for the Security Health Plan. Exhibit C is an organizational chart for the Marshfield Clinic.

Richard Leer, MD, President of the Marshfield Clinic and a family practice physician, still spends 20 percent of his time seeing patients; "This is part of our culture."

EXHIBIT C.
Organizational Chart, Marshfield Clinic

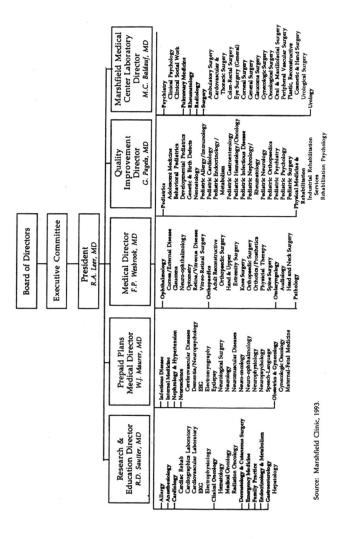

Source: Marshfield Clinic, 1993.

Finances. One of the unique aspects of Marshfield Clinic is that it traditionally has built up its financial reserves; it has not paid out all of its residual income after expenses in the form of physician compensation. For example, in fiscal year 1992 (ending September 30), the clinic had total assets of $177.5 million and equity of $73.8 million. Cash and short-term investments were $26.9 million. Ronald Pfannerstill, Director, Financial Affairs, said that the last time the clinic used its line of credit was in 1976.

Pfannerstill said that when he came to Marshfield in 1975, "The clinic was on a cash basis. We switched over to accrual." Wenzel noted that Pfannerstill has been a pioneer in installing cost accounting systems, and that Marshfield has used cost accounting since the late 1970s. "We can trace our costs to specific departments, physicians or a diagnosis."

Wenzel said that in the late 1970s the clinic recognized the need to begin to accumulate capital. (The clinic had a negative net worth in 1976.) "The president of the clinic agreed. We began with the proposal that the clinic hold back enough to cover one month's payroll. We painted some scenarios of what might go wrong and why we might need these monies. Some physicians referred to this as 'the Rib Mountain explosion' contingency fund. (Rib Mountain is a ski area near Wausau.) But, they bought the idea, and this allowed us to begin to strengthen our balance sheet."

Dr. Leer said that Marshfield's strong financial position makes the clinic more attractive to physicians. "They see us as financially stable."

Patient revenues in 1992 were $231.7 million. Of this, $142.8 million accounted for salaries and wages (all employees including physicians), and $14.5 million was spent on scientific research and education. Net earnings were $7.7 million. Exhibit B, presented earlier, includes a summary of revenues, expenses and earnings for 1988 through 1992.

St. Joseph's Hospital

St. Joseph's Hospital is the flagship of the Ministry Corporation, Sisters of the Sorrowful Mother, based in Milwaukee.

St. Joseph's is a busy and successful hospital with a large drawing area; 40 percent of the patients come from beyond 50 miles of Marshfield. Admissions have increased from 16,900 in 1988 to 17,700 in the last fiscalyear ending September 30, 1992. Patient days have increased from 125,500 in 1988 to 128,700 in 1992. This is in a period of declining hospital admissions and inpatient days in most parts of the US. Exhibit D summarizes several volume and financial indicators for the past five years.

EXHIBIT D.
Key Indicators, St. Joseph's Hospital
1988-1992 (Year-ending September 30)

Indicator	1988	1989	1990	1991	1992
Total Operating Revenue	$85,876,322	$97,969,530	$119,408,145	$129,188,678	$141,988,495
Expense	$81,454,551	$91,972,554	$106,309,276	$117,698,034 *	$129,765,125 *
Net Income	$5,766,098	$6,627,251	$14,590,439	$16,205,618 **	$17,179,237
Patient Days	125,532	124,027	127,779	127,060	128,708
Admissions	16,869	16,242	16,864	17,258	17,692
Average LOS (days)	7.44	7.64	7.58	7.36	7.27

Payor Mix (Based on Patient Days)					
Medicare	48.9%	47.5%	48.7%	48.6%	50.7%
Medicaid	7.9	7.8	7.7	8.0	9.5
Blue Cross	3.5	3.3	3.7	3.8	4.4
HMO	12.9	12.3	11.0	9.9	8.5
Commercial	23.3	26.0	26.0	26.7	24.1
Other	3.5	3.0	2.9	3.0	2.8

* Bad debt included in Expenses not Total Operating Revenue.
** Includes $1,923,934 extraordinary gain on recognition of deferred third-party payor reimbursement.
Source: St. Joseph's Hospital, April, 1993.

Total hospital revenues were $142 million in fiscal year 1992. Net income was $17.7 million for this same period.

Michael Schmidt, President and CEO of St. Joseph Hospital, noted that because of the clinic's ownership of radiology, out-patient surgery and other ancillary services, the hospital's outpatient revenues are around 10 percent of total revenues, well below hospital industry averages. "But, the clinic needs these revenues to help finance its system, and we certainly benefit from what they do and their success."

Schmidt said that the loss of certain revenue sources is "OK as long as we focus on increasing the size of the pie to make up for the fact that we are getting a smaller share."

From a pricing viewpoint, Schmidt said that St. Joseph's is in the middle of the pack in comparison with all Wisconsin hospitals. "But we are higher than Wausau." He said that the hospital's management team is working hard to reduce costs.

Relationships Between Marshfield Clinic, Ministry Corporation and St. Joseph's Hospital

Wenzel said that when he came to the clinic in the 1950s, the clinic and the hospital had a "love-hate" relationship. At one time the hospital tried to hire its own pathologists and radiologists.

He continued, "Over the past few years we have developed a much closer relationship with the hospital and its parent, the Ministry Corporation. In fact, we recently jointly purchased a clinic in Rice Lake. We also signed a letter of intent to purchase and operate a hospital in a small town in the northern part of the state. And I am sure we will pursue other ventures together in the future."

A Joint Conference Committee involving hospital and clinic leadership meets weekly. There is a monthly meeting of key Marshfield Clinic physicians and managers with individuals from the Ministry Corporation. According to Wenzel, "This monthly meeting is where some serious business takes place regarding the future of the two organizations."

Dr. Leer explained that when the Joint Conference Committee started, it dealt with a lot of detail. "Now we are really focusing on strategic issues."

He also said, "The Ministry Corporation's regional hospital system doesn't mesh geographically very well with the Marshfield Clinic's service area. But, this has the advantage of bringing us in contact with physicians whom we wouldn't otherwise meet. It improves communication and some of these doctors are in our health plan panel."

The Health Plan

Marshfield Clinic established the Greater Marshfield Community Health Plan, an HMO, in 1971. The plan was originally a partnership among the clinic, Blue Cross/Blue Shield United of Wisconsin and St. Joseph's Hospital.

The health plan fell on hard times leading to dissolution of the partnership in 1986, with Marshfield Clinic buying out the partners. Renamed Security Health Plan, the HMO had 65,000 subscribers in central and northern Wisconsin in 1993.

According to William Maurer, MD, Medical Director for the HMO and former president of the clinic, "The plan was community rated until 1986, and this caused serious problems with adverse selection. Once we switched to experience rating after we took the plan over, profitability improved. In fact, we now make $7 million to $8 million per year on the plan."

There are 800 providers in the panel; this means that more than 400 participating physicians and other health professionals are from outside the Marshfield Clinic. These providers are paid on a discounted fee-for-service basis. However, according to Dr. Maurer, payments to outside providers represent only two to three percent of all physician costs associated with the plan, and lack of control over utilization has not been a problem.

In early 1993, the Security Health Plan accounted for one quarter of the revenues of the clinic.

Regional Network Development

Wenzel said that in 1970 the Marshfield Clinic had a single location. The first relationship with another community occurred in the mid-1970s. "The town of Mosinee (25 miles northeast of Marshfield) came to us after their physician left. By coincidence, a physician came to us looking for a practice in a small town, and we recruited him to fill this spot." (Mosinee became an official part of the Marshfield Clinic in 1976.)

Three years earlier, a physician in Stratford, 10 miles north of Marshfield, died, and a Marshfield Clinic doctor began serving people in the area on a part-time basis. This led to the eventual location of the first official Marshfield regional center in Stratford.

Wenzel said that the clinic's philosophy in the 1970s was not to go anywhere unless local people asked the clinic to come in. However, in the late 1970s that policy changed, and Marshfield Clinic began to more aggressively develop new regional centers and satellites. "If we were going to operate a multispecialty clinic, we needed a primary care base to support it." In early 1993, the clinic had 22 regional care centers and satellites; these are identified in Exhibit E. Exhibit F lists the outlying clinics along with the year they were established. (Four of the outlying centers provide specialty services as well as primary care.)

EXHIBIT E.
Location of Marshfield Clinic's Regional Centers, 1993

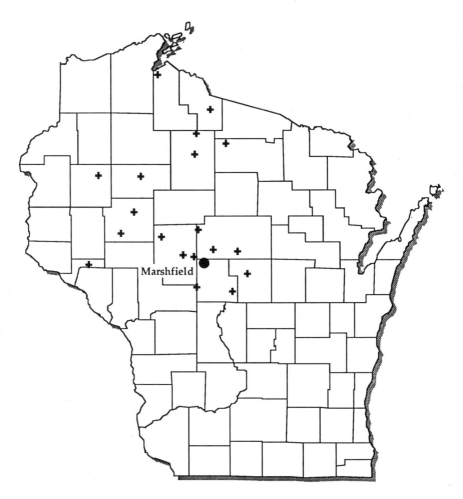

Marshfield

Source: Marshfield Clinic, 1993.

EXHIBIT F.
Marshfield Clinic Regional Centers and Year Established

Center	Year
Stratford	1973
Mosinee	1976
Ladysmith	1977
Greenwood	1978
Stanley	1978
Loyal	1983
Colby	1984
Abbotsford	1986
Thorp	1986
Chippewa Falls	1987
Durand	1987
Stevens Point*	1988
Mercer	1989
Minocqua/Woodruff	1989
Park Falls	1989
Phillips	1989
Ashland*	1991
Rice Lake	1991
Wisconsin Rapids*	1991
Pittsville	1992
Cornell	1993

* Single specialty sites.

Wenzel also noted that there was a relationship between the development of Marshfield's emphasis on primary care and the birth and development of the Greater Marshfield Community Health Plan in 1971. "At first it was believed that the health plan could be staffed by Marshfield Clinic physicians only. When we found there was great demand in the area from people interested in joining the plan, it was obvious that other primary care providers would have to be added. That led to affiliations, first with the health plan, and later on, with the clinic.

The clinic found the need to establish primary care as the health plan moved into rural Wisconsin."

Dr. Wesbrook recalled, "Seven or eight years ago we made a decision about allocating resources. The choice was between primary care centers in rural areas versus expanding here at our home base. We get an average of one request a week from physicians or small groups wanting to affiliate. I am glad we made the decision we did."

Dr. Leer, the clinic president, said that Marshfield's experience indicates that an organization can successfully integrate primary care physicians who come from a solo practitioner background.

When acquiring these rural practices, Marshfield Clinic purchases the assets and makes the physicians members of the clinic. Marshfield does not pay a premium for goodwill.

In addition to the rural practice sites, 80 Marshfield physicians regularly visit other communities to provide consulting services. This is a rapidly growing service.

Physician Mix/Compensation

Approximately one-quarter of the physicians on the staff of the Marshfield Clinic (including the outlying locations) are in primary care. This proportion has grown steadily over the past two decades.

Wenzel said, "I do recall debates back in the early 1960s about whether we should have family physicians. It caught on in the late 1960s, and now the Department of Family Medicine is very strong."

In general, Marshfield pays primary care physicians more than they would probably make in private practice settings. Specialists generally earn less than they would elsewhere.

Dr. Wesbrook, who provides staff support for the compensation committee, said that the committee is made up of four physicians, each elected for a three-year term. "Salaries range from $110,000 to $425,000 (one individual). A few are over $300,000 but most are in the $150,000 to $250,000 range."

Dr. Maurer noted that physician salaries were differentiated based on specialty beginning in 1980. "I think it was a mistake to cave in to a limited number of specialists on this. It started small and has continued to grow. It began with a four percent premium for 'what you put on the books' and continued to grow from there. I liked the old system a lot better."

In terms of financial subsidies for primary care physicians, Dr. Wesbrook said, "I think that is the wrong way to look at it. They are a necessary component of an integrated system. If the financial performance of an organization is to be optimized, it is necessary for some functions to be sub-optimized. That's the way systems work. Organizations who talk about a subsidy aren't going to have primary care physicians around for long."

Marshfield Clinic has a policy of not laying off physicians. Dr. Wesbrook said, "If times become tough, we will all take pay cuts, but there will be no layoffs." He went on to say, "There is a lot of flexibility to do primary care among our staff. We have well developed systems for triaging patients, and if a specialist is light on patients, he or she can be involved in the initial contact with patients."

In terms of the clinic's ability to adjust its compensation system as times change, Dr. Leer said, "I think across the country you are going to see specialists' incomes cascade down. First the high rollers will get hit. This will be followed by those who are taking a lot of money out of single-specialty groups. Then it will hit other organizations like Marshfield. But, we will be able to adjust."

Other Aspects of Marshfield Clinic

Unique culture. Dr. Maurer said that bringing in new physicians "is like selling a religion. People are enthused about the culture and collegiality here."

Physicians joining Marshfield are encouraged to perform research, publish and teach. Marshfield physicians publish over 100 articles per year in scholarly medical journals. The clinic spends several million dollars per year in funding research and educational programs.

The clinic has several messengers who deliver mail and medical records throughout the building; internal distribution of messages takes no more than 30 minutes. Rapid communication and quick access to medical records is part of the Marshfield culture. (The medical records department for the clinic also handles medical records for the hospital.)

One of the unique aspects of Marshfield is its salary system. For example, an equal salary system was in effect from 1954 through 1980, until recruiting pressures from certain specialists forced a change. As noted earlier, physician salaries at Marshfield fall within a narrower range compared with most multispecialty medical staffs or group practices.

The so-called monthly "town meetings" of shareholders, usually attended by two-thirds of the clinic's 300 directors, are also unique in terms of the interest they generate. These meetings are videoconferenced to several outlying locations so that physicians in these regional centers can participate.

Another unique aspect of the Marshfield culture is that physicians park in the remote parking lots, freeing up space for patients to park their cars near the clinic.

Research and education. The clinic has 40 residents in training at any point in time. Nearly all of the research and education is coordinated through the Marshfield Medical Research Foundation, which is a division of the clinic. This change from independent not-for-profit status to being part of the clinic occurred October 1, 1990.

Continuous quality improvement. Wenzel said that the clinic has established a quality council but is moving slowly. "CQI is just common sense. Doing things over, or doing too much, is expensive, and we want to improve our processes."

Dr. Leer noted that the clinic has "studied CQI to death. We have money in the budget for some projects and training. We have a quality council and are prepared to do just-in-time training. The hospital is ahead of us."

Robert De Vita, Executive Director, reports that Marshfield Clinic has been accepted into a network of 50 health care organizations to share the results of their quality improvement efforts. He noted that the clinic has developed process study teams internally and carried out specific projects in areas like scheduling of the cardiac cath lab.

Outcomes measurement. Dr. Leer said that Marshfield has been gathering data on outcomes from coronary care and surgery. "We look at this annually, and participate in a national study."

Information systems. The clinic upgraded its computer systems in 1991. In early 1993, eight of the 22 regional sites were on the system, which has 2,400 terminals. Clinical and financial information is available on an on-line basis and provides real-time results of many tests and procedures.

The clinic information system will require a doubling of the size of the mainframe computer, and will involve $4 million for hardware and upgrades to the present system. (This is not the total cost of the new system.) The information system staff at Marshfield Clinic includes 82 people with 35 to 40 of those directly involved in system development.

St. Joseph's Hospital and Marshfield Clinic have separate data processing systems. Mike Schmidt of the hospital said, "In the future we need a centralized data base. We need to connect up referring physicians, the clinic and the hospital, and even nursing homes. I call this 'connectivity.'" He went on, "The hospital intends to spent $10 to $12 million over the next two years to replace and improve our data base and information system."

Robert De Vita said the clinic is talking seriously with Ministry Corporation (the parent of St. Joseph's Hospital) about revamping and inter-connecting the information systems of the two organizations. "We need to be able to connect the 'Tower of Babel.' The new system will include clinical information and the demographic characteristics of patients. It is all part of our ability to measure outcomes." When asked what this would cost, he said, "I don't have a firm estimate, but I know it will be several million dollars over the next few years, and this is on top of what the hospital plans to spend."

Malpractice insurance coverage. Marshfield Clinic is self insured for malpractice, and this process saved an estimated $5 million in the past year. Reed Hall said that the self insurance plan has $11 million in reserve. "Another advantage of being self insured is that department heads and others take the whole matter of risk management and quality control more seriously."

Laboratories. Marshfield Clinic operates several laboratories including a joint venture laboratory with the hospital, a reference laboratory that provides services to hospitals over a large multi-state area and a veterinarian laboratory (off campus).

Major Accomplishments

Dr. Leer identified four major accomplishments of the past 10 or 15 years:

- Acquisition of regional centers; building rural referral network.

- Governance and communication among physicians.

- Capital to finance technology, equipment and information systems.

- Commitment to education and research.

Ronald Pfannerstill said that the clinic ownership structure and the monthly shareholder meetings have meant that Marshfield physicians have become knowledgeable about finances. "Physicians here understand the difference between accrual and cash accounting, debt service ratios, current ratios, and other measures of financial performance."

Wenzel cited several accomplishments. "We have improved our financial position dramatically. We have built a rural referral network that covers the region and have added a subsequent number of primary care physicians to our clinic. We are working more closely with the Ministry Corporation. We have an HMO, and this is giving us experience with capitation. We are very well positioned for the future, especially if we have some form of managed competition."

According to Wenzel, the clinic is viewed by many residents of the area as being "pricey." "However," Wenzel said, "it is short sighted to only look at episodic care at the clinic and hospital; this is far different from what it costs to provide the total health care for a defined population."

He went on, "Through our relationship with the hospital we have virtually eliminated duplication of high-cost equipment and services. We are saving a substantial sum by being self insured. Our interest payments are lower because of our tax-exempt status. Salaries of physicians, especially specialists, are well below national averages. We have a steady patient flow and don't add physicians until the patient load justifies it; we aren't over staffed. Our peer review system, and collegiality, tends to drastically reduce inappropriate and unnecessary care. All this adds up to being cost effective. As we move more into capitation, we should do very well."

Lessons Learned

Fritz Wenzel identified several lessons learned:

- The patient must always be number one.

- It is important to recruit high quality physicians and a top-notch management team.

- The group must have visionary leadership at both the physician and non-physician level. You must be able to tolerate ambiguity, and be optimistic; there is no place for pessimism.

- The democratic form of governance has served Marshfield Clinic well.

- Establishing strong ties with the hospital and its parent corporation has been a long and arduous process, but this effort is now beginning to pay off.

- Establishment of a regional system is playing a key role in the success and development of the clinic.

- Communications and up-front honesty among the leaders of the clinic is critical.

Mike Schmidt, with the hospital, offered these three lessons learned from his perspective:

(1) Both organizations — the clinic and hospital — need to be successful; it won't work if one does well and the other does not.

(2) We can be better together; we don't have to fight over turf.

(3) Don't be afraid to look at the paradigm shift in health care; we can't be successful in a capitated environment without a close relationship.

Bob De Vita said there are three important lessons that he has learned from the Marshfield experience:

- Own as much of your referral network as possible. This doesn't mean that everyone has to work for you, although this is OK, but you must have economic ties with physicians in the network.

- Control the financing — the health plan — so the organization can take risks.

- Never lose sight of your mission, and it had better be customer driven.

Issues for the Future

Can a large professional group continue to be governed in a democratic fashion? Will the physician leadership have the strength and courage to face the challenges, both medical and economic, of the 1990s? Can Marshfield prove the value of coordinated care? These were issues raised by several Marshfield physicians and administrators.

De Vita identified these issues:

- Can we keep up with the pace of health care reform?

- Can we begin to think differently and do things differently? For example, can we adjust our physician compensation system to reflect the impact of a capitated payment system?

- Can we avoid the pressure to compete in destructive ways? We would prefer managed collaboration. But, if we are forced into competing, we can do that too.

Marshfield Clinic will face increased competition from large clinics located on its periphery. The Mayo Clinic, Duluth Clinic and Gundersen Clinic in La Crosse may become more competitive. Much depends on health care reform and the shape of the regions drawn for providing services.

---

* Fritz Wenzel and his staff organized the interviews and provided much of the data for this case study; our thanks to Fritz and all of the others at the Marshfield Clinic and St. Joseph's Hospital who contributed to this effort.

Case Study #4

CARLE CLINIC ASSOCIATION/
CARLE FOUNDATION HOSPITAL
Urbana, Illinois

— Persons Interviewed —

Kenneth Bash, Chief Administrative Officer, Carle Clinic Association
Doran Dunaway, Associate Administrator, Information Systems
Michael Fritz, President and CEO, Carle Foundation
Terry Hatch, MD, Assistant Vice President, Educational Services,
    Carle Foundation
Robert Hendrickson, Associate Administrator, Financial Services,
    Carle Clinic Association
B. Smith Hopkins, MD, retired, Carle Clinic Association
Orin Ireland, Vice President and Chief Financial Officer, Carle Foundation
C. Carleton King, Associate Administrator, Carle Clinic Association
    and Executive Director, Health Alliance Medical Plans
Gregory Lykins, Vice Chairman, Carle Foundation Board
Carol McClure, Manager of Benefits Services, University of Illinois
Terry Noonan, MD, Chairman, Carle Clinic Board of Governors
Robert Parker, MD, Medical Director, Carle Clinic Association,
    Vice President, Medical Services, Carle Foundation
John Pollard, MD, Chief Executive Officer, Carle Clinic Association
Thomas Schrepfer, MD, Vice Chairman, Carle Clinic Board of Governors
Edra Scofield, Director of Marketing and Planning,
    Carle Clinic Association
Robert Scully, MD, past Chairman, Carle Clinic Board of Governors
Dennis Sims, Director of Finance, Carle Clinic Association
Kenneth Waltsgott, Director of Human Resources, Super Value
Kenneth Weiss, MD, Head, Department of Surgery,
    Carle Clinic Association

April, 1993

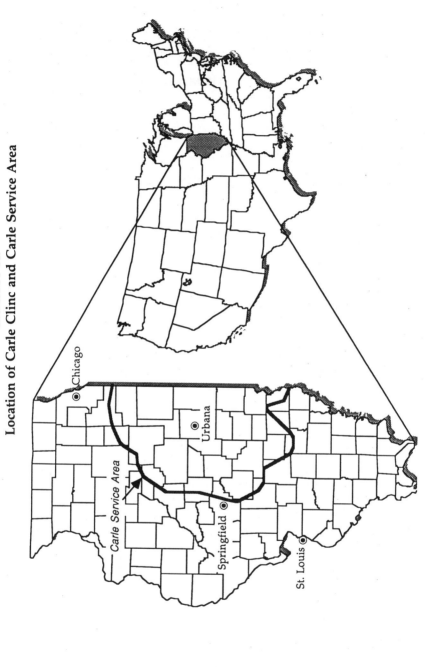

EXHIBIT A.

Location of Carle Clinc and Carle Service Area

CARLE CLINIC ASSOCIATION/ CARLE FOUNDATION HOSPITAL
Urbana, Illinois

The Carle Clinic Association is a 240-physician multispeciality clinic. The Carle Foundation Hospital is a 288-bed acute care facility located immediately adjacent to the clinic in Urbana.

The Urbana Market Area

The region. Located in Urbana (Champaign County), the Carle Clinic has a service area that covers a 90-mile radius. Exhibit A shows the location of Urbana and Champaign County within the State of Illinois and highlights the Carle Clinic service area.

The clinic's primary service area has an estimated population of 1.1 million; however, 49 percent of the clinic's patients originate within Champaign County which has a population of around 250,000. The University of Illinois, with 17,000 employees and 36,000 students, is the dominant economic force in the area.

The University of Illinois medical school in Urbana/Champaign provides training for 240 students in both MD and MD/PhD programs. Carle Clinic and Carle Hospital are the primary teaching sites for this program. Carle Clinic and Carle Hospital offer post-graduate residency programs in family practice, internal medicine, colon and rectal surgery and oral surgery.

Champaign-Urbana is 135 miles south of Chicago. St. Louis is 160 miles southwest of Urbana. Springfield, 90 miles west, is home of the Southern Illinois University medical school.

Competition in the Champaign-Urbana area. The Carle Clinic's major competitor is the Christie Clinic with 90 physicians. The Christie Clinic also owns Personal Care, an HMO with 35,600 members.

In addition to the two clinics, there are approximately 30 private practice physicians in the Champaign-Urbana area and another 18 physicians affiliated with the University of Illinois student health center.

Carle Clinic's market penetration within Champaign-Urbana was 34 percent, and 14 percent throughout the remainder of the 90-mile service area. Edra Scofield, Director of Marketing and Planning, Carle Clinic Association, estimates that approximately 20 percent of the physicians in the area beyond Champaign-Urbana are associated with the Carle Clinic.

In 1980, there were five hospitals in the Champaign-Urbana area; there were two survivors in 1993. The Carle Foundation Hospital is described later. The second largest hospital in the area, Covenant (the merged product of two hospitals, each which held approximately 33 percent market share), has 280 beds; however, this hospital had 43 percent of the Champaign County market in 1990, compared with 30 percent for Carle Foundation Hospital. Because of its close identification with the Carle Clinic, the Carle Foundation Hospital draws a higher proportion of its patients from a much larger geographic area.

History of the Carle Clinic

Early history — the Great Depression through World War II. The Rogers-Davison Clinic was founded in 1931 by Thomas Rogers, MD, and Hugh Davison, MD, two Mayo-trained physicians whose goal was to establish a new multispecialty group practice modeled after the Mayo Clinic.

Although several attempts were made in the 1920s to capitalize on a bequest from the Carle family to build and sustain a hospital in Urbana, these efforts failed in 1930. When Drs. Rogers and Davison came to Urbana there was no hospital; however, the hospital building provided the first location for the Rogers-Davison Clinic.

By 1935, Drs. Rogers and Davison had been joined by six other Mayo-trained physicians to form the nucleus of what has become one of the large group practices in the country. A year later, in 1936, the group formed the Carle Hospital Association, a not-for-profit organization capitalized at $5,000, to operate the hospital. The clinic then leased space from the hospital.

The naming of the new facility was a fairly simple matter. . . The community had become familiar with the Carle name; this family of pioneers had long been recognized as public benefactors in Urbana. Thus, Carle Memorial Hospital was a popular and fortunate choice. At the same time, Dr. Davison's name and mine were quite unknown in Champaign-Urbana. Putting our names together as a medical entity was an ethical means of gaining public recognition (from *Carle: Concept and Growth*, a book by J. C. Thomas Rogers, page 34).

B. Smith Hopkins, MD, came to the Carle Clinic prior to World War II when there were 12 physicians on the staff. He said the number shrunk to four doctors during the war. When the war ended, six of the original eight founders returned to Carle. "It was touch and go during the war whether the Carle Clinic would make it."

The changes of the 1950s. Dr. Hopkins said that up until the 1950s all of the clinic's physicians, other than the six partners, were salaried employees. "But, a number of us were uneasy about this arrangement. We thought we should have more of a role in developing the clinic. In the mid-1950s we were able to achieve some change in our status, including the election of three salaried physicians to the Board of Governors (total of nine including the original six physicians). Over the next few years we were able to achieve an increasing degree of participation in the management and governance of the clinic."

Many at the Carle Clinic believe that decisions to broaden the ownership and management base represented critical success factors in the subsequent growth of the clinic.

The past 14 years. John Pollard, MD, a cardiologist who also has an MBA degree, became the Chief Executive Officer of the clinic in 1979. According to a number of physicians at Carle, Pollard is the person most responsible for establishing the present system of branches, bringing in family practice, developing the health plan, and generally making sure that Carle Clinic continued to be successful.

One of the members of the Carle Clinic management team said, "Three of Dr. Pollard's initiatives have turned out to be extremely important for the future of the clinic. These were the addition of family practice, the branches and development of the health plan (all discussed later in this case study). All of these decisions ran against the prevailing culture of the clinic at the time, and all were risky."

Dr. Pollard, like all Carle physician administrators, maintains a medical practice; he spends 20 percent of his time seeing patients. "Dr. Parker, the Medical Director and I are the only exceptions to the rule that physician administrators should spend at least 50 percent of their time on patient care."

Indicators of growth. Exhibit B shows patient visits and revenues for the Carle Clinic from 1988 through 1992.

EXHIBIT B.
Trends in Patient Visits and Revenues,
Carle Clinic, 1988-1992

Year	Patient Contacts	Revenues ($ Millions)
1988	545,450	$85
1989	602,800	86
1990	585,900	101
1991	571,500	114
1992	594,900	119

Source: Carle Clinic internal records, May, 1993.

The clinic grew from 33 physicians in 1960, to 67 in 1970. By 1980, the number of physicians had reached 108. The figure for 1990 was 209, and for early 1993, the number reached 240.

During this same period revenues increased dramatically. In 1960, net revenues of the Carle Clinic were $2.4 million. In 1988, revenues were $85 million. By 1992, clinic revenues had reached $119 million.

According to Edra Scofield, the demand for physician services at Carle continues to exceed the supply. "If we are going to increase our revenues and market penetration, we are going to have to add more doctors."

Carle Foundation Hospital

The Carle Foundation Hospital (288 beds) is the largest hospital in Champaign County; Covenant Hospital was larger, but in April, 1992, it combined its Champaign and Urbana campuses and downsized from 449 to 280 beds. Patient discharges from the two hospitals in 1992 were almost identical — 14,000 each.

The occupancy rate for the Carle Hospital was 69.5 percent in 1991. This was significantly higher than any hospital in the service area.

The Carle Foundation Hospital provides a broad array of services to residents of its service area. Michael Fritz, President and CEO, said that major organ transplants are the only procedure not performed at the hospital. "We do everything else," he said.

Fritz said that one of the major advantages of Carle is that there is little or no duplication of clinical services and equipment. "When you don't duplicate you remove a major source of contention between physicians and a hospital." He cited two other advantages of operating a hospital as part of the Carle system:

- We can agree to do things more quickly and get them done.

- The hospital has been financially successful, especially over the past three or four years. This is despite the fact that the clinic operates several of the most profitable activities typically offered by a hospital; for example, laboratory and radiology.

Fritz also said that the hospital does not have to worry about physicians getting upset and threatening to take their business elsewhere. "This frees us up to think more strategically rather than constantly putting out fires."

The financial position of the Foundation (including the hospital and several other entities) was strong with $208 million in assets as of June 30, 1992. Fund balances (net worth) were just under $74 million. Long-term debt was $109 million.

Total revenues of the Foundation, coming primarily from the hospital, were just over $90 million in the year ended June 30, 1992. Net income for this period was $8.8 million.

In terms of payor mix, in 1992 the hospital received 36 percent of its net revenues from Medicare and 31 percent from commercial and private pay sources. Just over 20 percent of the hospital's revenues came from CarleCare. Medicaid represented 10 percent of hospital revenues.

Administratively, the department heads of the clinic are also the department heads for the hospital; this reduces redundancy. Robert Parker, MD, Medical Director, Carle Clinic Association, said, "All the clinical, risk management and related matters for both the hospital and clinic report to me. I have two bosses — the board of governors of the clinic and board of trustees of the hospital."

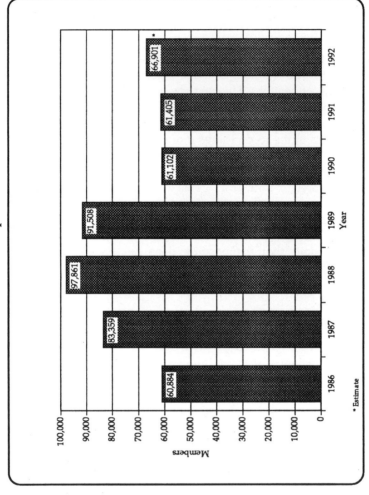

EXHIBIT C.
HMO Membership At Year End

From a cost viewpoint, Fritz said that the data he has reviewed indicate that the Carle Foundation Hospital is "in the middle of pack" among larger Illinois hospitals.

Health Plans

Carle Clinic owns and operates the Health Alliance Medical Plans, Inc. (HAMP), a for-profit stock insurance company. CarleCare, a for-profit HMO, had 68,000 members in 400 groups in early 1993. The Health Alliance PPO, with 3,000 participants, represents a second major line of business. Exhibit C shows the trend in CarleCare enrollment over the past few years. HAMP's revenues in 1992 were $87 million, mainly from the HMO.

Carle originally formed a management company in 1980 to manage what was then a not-for-profit HMO. The HMO was converted to for-profit status in 1988, and HAMP was formed in November, 1989 in order to be able to offer PPO products; the offering of such products required a broad insurance license from the State of Illinois.

In addition HAMP administers the clinic and foundation self-insurance plans for employees and physicians. The HAMP board is the clinic board of governors.

When the HMO was started, the Champaign-Urbana health care marketplace was dominated by indemnity insurance. The Christie Clinic had started an HMO, but other than this organization, there was little in the way of managed care. Therefore, concern about competing with health plan customers was not given much thought. Kenneth Bash, Chief Administrative Officer, Carle Clinic Association, said, "We viewed the patients and payors as our customers; not the health plans. People had complete freedom of choice back in those days, and we were concentrating on getting their business."

As shown on Exhibit C, CarleCare peaked at 97,900 members in 1988. According to C. Carleton King, Associate Administrator, Carle Clinic Association and Executive Director, HAMP, this was at a time when underwriting standards were not adequate; these standards were subsequently increased and several groups were dropped from the plan in 1989 and 1990. In addition, Carle had entered into joint venture arrangements outside its service area that proved to be unworkable. The major reduction in membership resulted from a contraction of the service area. With the reduced membership, the HMO has been profitable, generating close to $10 million in profits in its last year.

Kenneth Bash said that Carle has not made a large out-of-pocket investment in getting the HMO off and running. "We had the delivery system in place, and we never kept track of the administrative costs of starting the HMO; it was just another part of our job. Therefore, the incremental costs of getting into the health plan business was not large, probably no more than $1 million."

King said, "There are two issues involved in running a profitable HMO — underwriting and management, especially controlling utilization. When we started the HMO, the underwriting criteria were too loose, we ended up with a poor risk pool, and we lost money. It doesn't matter how good a job of managing you do, if you have a poor risk pool you won't make money with an HMO."

Currently, when the Carle Clinic provides services to the HMO, the clinic is at risk; it is paid on a capitated basis. King said that within CarleCare, less than 10 percent of the expenses are paid to out-of-system providers. (The proportion of non-Carle physicians was substantially higher when enrollment peaked in 1988.)

King said there are several ways in which the Carle Clinic and Carle Foundation Hospital contribute to the profitability of the health plan:

(1)   Continuum of care. "This means you can match patients' needs with the most appropriate level of care."

(2)   Emphasis on outpatient care. "Carle has a tradition of outpatient care that goes back a long ways. This is the cost effective way to do things."

(3)   Hub and spoke branching system. "This is an efficient way to provide primary care services and use specialists appropriately."

(4)   Lower overhead. "The health plan can share the costs of certain services, such as personnel and purchasing."

(5)   Greater use of physician extenders, or "collaborative practices."

(6)   Centralized leadership and governance. "This reduces competition and gives everyone the same sense of direction."

Relative to physician extenders, King noted that under the present payment system it is often difficult to get these professionals paid for the services they provide. Therefore, there is less incentive to use them. "But, capitation will change all of this. I see them playing a much bigger role in the future as we move into a capitated system."

King said that the Carle system may be somewhat inefficient because of the nature of a multispecialty practice. "There is a tendency for physicians to do more extensive workups. Therefore, the quality advantage of the clinic might work against us from the perspective of a health plan or payor."

Over the past five years, CarleCare has represented between 35 and 42 percent of Carle Clinic's revenues.

Governance/Relationship Among Various Organizations Within Carle

Exhibit D shows an organizational chart for the major entities making up the Carle integrated health care system. The major elements are The Carle Foundation, which owns and operates the hospital and a number of other entities, and the Carle Clinic Association. This exhibit also shows the reporting relationship of the Joint Policy Council and Joint Administrative Group, and the years each of the subsidiaries began operations.

Carle Foundation. The Foundation owns all the real estate of the organization, including the clinic, and leases these back to the various entities.

Since the clinic is not in a position to accumulate capital, the Foundation acts as the source of credit, or the bank, for the rest of the entities. One person explained, "The Foundation is the landlord, and the hospital and clinic pay rent."

The Foundation board consists of six community representatives, five Carle Clinic physicians and the Foundation CEO (Michael Fritz).

Carle Clinic Board of Governors. New physicians may become shareholders of the clinic after two years of practice at Carle and approval of three-quarters of the associates. In 1993, there were 165 shareholders.

EXHIBIT D.

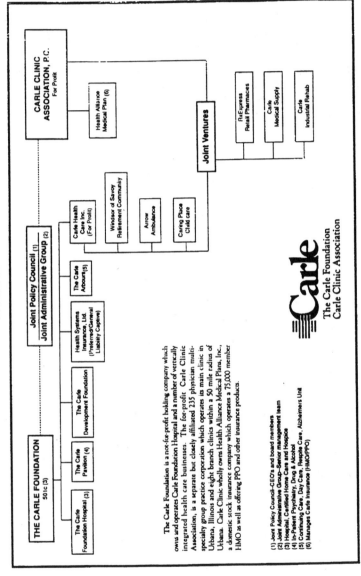

The Carle Foundation is a not-for-profit holding company which owns and operates Carle Foundation Hospital and a number of vertically integrated health care businesses. The for-profit Carle Clinic Association, is a separate but closely affiliated 235 physician multi-specialty group practice corporation which operates its main clinic in Urbana, Illinois and eight branch clinics within a 50 mile radius of Urbana. Carle Clinic wholly owns Health Alliance Medical Plans, Inc., a domestic stock insurance company which operates a 75,000 member HMO as well as offering PPO and other insurance products.

(1) Joint Policy Council–CEO's and board members
(2) Joint Administrative Group–Senior management team
(3) Hospital, Certified Home Care and Hospice
(4) In-Patient Psychiatry, Drug & Alcohol
(5) Continuing Care, Day Care, Respite Care, Alzheimers Unit
(6) Manages Carle Insurance (HMO/PPO)

The Carle Foundation
Carle Clinic Association

The policy-making body of the clinic is its Board of Governors, consisting of six physicians elected by the shareholders for staggered three-year terms.

Joint Policy Council. Members of this council include the six physicians who are on the Carle Clinic's Board of Governors and the executive committee of the Foundation. This group focuses on strategic issues facing Carle. The Joint Policy Council has no legal authority and the two boards act independently.

Joint Administrative Group. This is the coordinating body between the clinic, hospital and other entities within the Carle Foundation. The group meets weekly. Kenneth Bash noted that although the group has no authority, the planning carried out is important to the organization.

Orin Ireland, Vice President and Chief Financial Officer, Carle Foundation, said, "The two organizations — the clinic and hospital — have a long history of working together (back to the 1930s), and a level of trust has built up. There are several areas waiting to be integrated, but regulatory and legal uncertainties keep us from doing it."

Compensation

Kenneth Bash said that the Carle Clinic compensation pool is based on net revenues less expenses for the year. Overhead for Carle is around 59 percent of net revenues; therefore, the physician pool would typically be around 41 percent.

The three elements considered in dividing the compensation pool are:

- *Association factor — 25 percent.* This is similar to seniority. After four years a physician receives a full share of this portion of the compensation pool.

- *Production factor — 70 percent.* This is based on a system of targets for specific specialties, with compensation being based on whether a physician is over or under the norm.

- *Board factor — five percent.* The Board of Governors allocates a portion of these dollars to department heads for distribution to physicians in each department. There are no predetermined criteria; it is up to the department chairperson. Equal distributions to each physician are discouraged, and the Board of Governors retains ultimate authority over physician incomes.

Bash said that there is a seven-to-one range for physician compensation, but that 80 percent of the salaries are within a three-to-one range (the highest salary is three times the lowest). Salaries are set at 80 percent of a physician's previous year's total compensation.

In recruiting new physicians, Bash said that salaries are generally established based on the market, and they are adjusted, as appropriate.

Dr. Pollard believes that future trends in the compensation of physicians will favor primary care. At the Carle Clinic, new primary care physicians earn $90,000 up to $110,000 plus fringe benefits. "The range is seven times as high and this is too much. However, salaries reflect the external environment. When the marketplace changes, our salaries will also shift."

Primary care physicians at Carle do not generally generate sufficient net income, after deductions for their share of overhead, to cover the salaries paid to them. The funds to make up this deficit come from the rest of the organization, including health plan and ancillary profits and the earnings of specialists. Thomas Schrepfer, MD, Vice Chairman, Carle Clinic Board of Governors, said, "The so-called subsidy is a two-way street. Primary care physicians keep the specialists busy."

The Emphasis on Family Practice and Branches

Family practice. Dr. Pollard said, "In 1975, it was hard to get in to see one of our physicians. We were busy and satisfied. The opinion of many specialists of family practice physicians was not high. But, we could see that people were flocking to family practice docs; they were voting with their feet. Some of us concluded that if we had some of these types of physicians it would help with the work load."

Dr. Pollard went on: "It was important for our staff to get to know the first family practice doctor and what he could do. This helped change minds about family practice. Right now, with 40 doctors, family practice is the largest and fastest growing department within the clinic."

Branches. According to Dr. Pollard, there are four kinds of branches:

- Main branch — Urbana.

- Primary care along with some specialists — Champaign and Southeast Urbana are examples.

- Family practice branches — These tend to be in small communities within a 20 to 30 mile radius of Urbana.

- Multispecialty branches — These are usually within 35 to 60 miles of Urbana; Carle has three of these types of branches. These branches are also referred to as "hubs."

Dr. Pollard said the first branch was started with pediatricians. "We started in a trailer in a shopping center in Mahomet, 20 miles from here. This clinic now has five family practice physicians and no pediatricians." He noted that most of the branches have been established by hiring new physicians, not by acquisition of existing medical practices.

The 10 branch clinics, the number of physicians in each and the year each branch was established are shown below:

Location	Number of Physicians	Year Established
Mahomet	4	1978
Rantoul	4	1980
Bloomington/Normal	20	1983
Champaign	15	1983
Danville	16	1983
Monticello	5	1985
Georgetown	1	1987
Mattoon & Charleston	5	1988
Southeast Urbana	2 + resident training	1989
Tuscola	1	1990

The clinic's strategic plan calls for the establishment of additional branches and for expansion of some of the hubs.

With respect to relationships with physicians in surrounding communities, Edra Scofield said, "I believe you either own the primary care physician's practice (and have them on salary) or have them tied to you through the health plan. If you don't do this you are vulnerable to losing them to competing organizations. It is risky in this environment to count on good will or friendships."

Kenneth Weiss, MD, Head, Department of Surgery, Carle Clinic Association, noted, "One of the secrets to the success of Carle is its primary care network. The only problem is the cost and the need to continually subsidize this network."

Branching and the health plan. Dr. Pollard said the health plan and branching strategies are interrelated. "For example, an employer in Danville wanted to be in our health plan, but we had no physicians in the area. This is one of the reasons we established a branch in Danville." The health plan is offered in all geographic areas where the clinic has physicians.

Carleton King agreed. "Managed care and branching strategies are synergistic." Dr. Schrepfer said, "The HMO, branches and our emphasis on family practice physicians is a tripod that has been very important to our success, and it represents a building block for the future."

Relationship of primary care physicians and specialists. Dr. Parker said that between 1931 and 1970, all of the physicians at Carle were specialists. In 1980, by contrast, between one quarter and one third of the Carle physicians were in primary care. "In 1990, I estimate that approximately half of the 240 physicians at Carle were in primary care."

Dr. Pollard said, "You tell me the size of the group or medical staff and I can pretty much tell you what the mix of specialties will be." He went on to say that within the Carle culture, if a specialist is not busy, he or she is usually willing to do some primary care. "Our physicians understand the need for this kind of flexibility."

Other Aspects of Carle Foundation and Carle Clinic

Corporate culture. Dr. Weiss said that the corporate cultures of the hospital and clinic are markedly different. "In the hospital, if the CEO tells a subordinate to do something, they do it. In the clinic, however, if the CEO tells one of the physicians to do something, he may argue vehemently against it. There is constant friction and a tug of war. You have more big egos and hidden agendas. There is more need for consensus building."

In comparing the cultures of the clinic and Foundation, Michael Fritz said they are different. "The Foundation operates more like a major corporation; it is management driven. The clinic is more democratic.

There is a lot of strength in the departments." He went on, "In the Foundation it takes us longer to make decisions, but we can hold them. The clinic makes decisions faster, but sometimes they can't hold them."

Continuous quality improvement. Dr. Parker said that the clinic and hospital spent much of 1991 developing a vision statement and values. In 1992, a Florida firm was hired to help develop the new quality improvement initiative. The clinic and hospital have a combined quality council. Dr. Parker added, "The National Demonstration Project organizations tended to bring physicians into the process later; we think this was a terrible mistake."

In early 1993, there were between 30 and 50 quality teams working. There have been 24 three-day courses offered, each attended by 22 Carle employees. All employees have gone through a three-hour "macro" course. All senior managers and board members have received more intensive training. Four teams of Carle staff members (three persons per team) have been trained and now teach the internal seminars on continuous quality improvement.

Information systems. One physician commented, "We are 'seamless' in the delivery of care but our computer systems are not."

Doran Dunaway, Associate Administrator, Information Systems (IS), said that Carle is revamping the hospital system to increase compatibility between the hospital and the clinic systems. They are also planning to install an order system for the lab, pharmacy and radiology. Once this is completed, physicians at all locations will be able to place orders for their patients on-site. This systems upgrade will also allow physicians to bring all patient information on line.

The estimated cost of the system upgrade will be $3.5 million with annual maintenance costing approximately 10-14 percent of the original cost each year ($350,000-$490,000/year). The hospital will be responsible for the cost of this upgrade. Carle Clinic has 75 people in the IS department, with 45-50 of those directly involved with systems development.

The current information system in place at Carle Clinic is based on the registration component. Registration involves capturing patient information and demographics during a patient's first visit to the clinic or hospital. Carle Clinic has 1.1 million active patients in its system.

Registration is also a common component in the information systems at the hospital and at the HMO. The clinic, hospital and HMO all have the ability to "register" a patient and to retrieve patient information through a common system. In addition, seven of the clinic's branches are linked into the Carle system. Doran Dunaway estimated that there are 1,000 on-line devices throughout the network.

The current information system also includes parts of the medical records, demographics and insurance information, as well as linking the pharmacy, lab and radiology. Dunaway referred to their system as the "electronic highway" through which all entities (clinic, hospital and HMO) can communicate.

Dunaway pointed out that there is a disproportionate amount of programming available for hospital use versus that available for clinic use. He explained that hospitals go to great lengths to track information for inpatients who may have had only one or two stays. On the other hand, he said that the volume of outpatient visits justifies the need to track those patients more closely.

Outcomes measurement. Carle does not presently have systems in place to measure medical outcomes. As noted in the 1991 strategic plan, "Thus, Carle cannot immediately demonstrate to major payors the superiority of the care it can offer to patients" (p. 15).

Carle Clinic will be using the medical records portion of the system to perform outcomes measurement in the next year and a half or so. They are still in the process of entering medical records into the system. The hospital has performed some CQI work, but it has only involved the cost component and not specifically looked at outcomes.

Malpractice insurance. Carle Foundation owns a captive malpractice insurance company, Health Systems Insurance, that was initially capitalized at $1.8 million. Half of the board members for this corporation are from the clinic and half are from the Foundation.

The liability insurance company saves Carle 25 to 30 percent annually on malpractice premiums; this represents a savings of $500,000 per year.

Use of mid-level providers and patient advisory nurses. Carle employs more than 70 nurse practitioners, physician assistants, and certified nurse mid-wives. According to Kenneth Bash, the clinic strongly believes that this type of collaborative approach is cost effective for patients and payors.

Carle patient advisory nurses (there are 35 on the team) provide a 24-hour, seven days a week telephone service responding to patient questions. Referring physicians may also use the service to schedule their patients with specialists. During an average month, the patient advisory nurses receive 12,000 incoming telephone calls from people in need of assistance. This system has been beneficial to the HMO by reducing the number of ER visits and to the Carle physicians by making their on call duties more tolerable. The system also benefits referring physicians by saving time and facilitating their patients' appointments.

Other health-related activities. The Carle Foundation owns and operates a host of other businesses including Carle Home Care, Carle Pavilion (a 46-bed psychiatric and chemical dependency hospital), Carle Arbours (a 240-bed skilled nursing facility located five miles from the hospital), and Windsor of Savoy (a 137-unit retirement living center). The Arrow Medical Services Division operates an emergency rescue service and related activities.

The Foundation and clinic operate three businesses as joint ventures:

(a) The Carle Industrial Rehabilitation program provides conditioning programs and placement activities to facilitate injured workers' re-entry into the work force.

(b) RxExpress is a retail pharmacy with seven locations consisting of pharmacies in the main branch in Urbana and at several other branch locations.

(c) Carle Medical Supply operates retail outlets for durable medical goods in Urbana and Mattson, Illinois.

Core Competencies

The 1991 strategic planning effort identified six core competencies for Carle:

- *Multidisciplinary care.* This relates to the multispecialty nature of the clinic.

- *Continuum of program competencies.*

- *Integrated delivery of care.*

- *Ability to transition health care in rural communities.* This relates to the hub and spoke branching system and use of outreach clinics by specialists.

- *Demonstrated excellence in health care.*

- *Ability to recruit and retain physicians.* According to several individuals, more physicians than ever are expressing interest in joining Carle.

Major Accomplishments/Success Factors

Dr. Pollard believes that the major benefits of the clinic are that it serves patients better, physicians stay current with changes in medical technology and the clinic setting offers physicians a reasonable lifestyle (e.g., less burden of being on-call, ability to take a vacation).

In terms of how he measures the success of Carle, Kenneth Bash cited three factors:

(1) *Innovation.* "We pioneered the use of nurse practitioners and physician assistants, and the use of patient advice nurses. This has dramatically reduced the number of after-hours calls to physicians."

(2) *Financial strength.* The Carle system is in a solid financial position, has a successful HMO and rewards physicians well.

(3) *Integration.* The Carle system has forward integration through its primary care branches and its HMO, and backward integration through rehabilitation, home health care services, psych and substance abuse, and the full continuum of long-term care housing and medical services described earlier.

Edra Scofield said that, in her opinion, the two major factors that have contributed to the success of Carle over the past decade have been the branches and the health plan.

Gregory Lykins, Vice Chairman, Carle Foundation Board, said that in the community Carle is viewed as a single entity. "People around here don't differentiate between the clinic and hospital. Carle — the whole entity — is viewed as being progressive and modern." He also believes that Carle is adept at changing with the rapidly shifting health care environment.

Kenneth Waltsgott, Director of Human Resources for Super Value, one of the largest employers in the Champaign-Urbana area with 1,000 employees, said that the quality of care provided by Carle is good. "We encourage second opinions, but our experience is that the diagnosis of a Carle physician is almost always correct and appropriate care has been specified."

Robert Scully, MD, past Chairman, Carle Board of Governors, indicated that there are five "secrets of success" for Carle:

(1) Carle really is a group practice. "Christie Clinic is organized as a group, but operates as a group of departments."

(2) The productivity of physicians is high. "The medical staff is made up of very hard workers."

(3) The majority of physicians think "group" rather than in terms of what is best for them individually.

(4) Access to tax-exempt capital is available through the Foundation. "Lots of organizations flounder because of lack of capital. We certainly wouldn't have branches without a source of real estate financing."

(5) Carle has excellent leadership. "Dr. Pollard has been an outstanding leader. You can't always plan on what you are going to have in the way of leadership; we have been fortunate."

According to the Foundation's 1992 bond prospectus (page A-22), "Branch development adds to the referral system utilizing the services of the main campus. This referral system is in large part responsible for the obligated group's (the hospital primarily) ability to maintain strong utilization in an era where the general trend among acute care providers is declining utilization."

Lessons Learned

Kenneth Bash cited several lessons learned:

*   Even though the Carle Clinic and Carle Foundation work together closely, and have for many years, it is important to have formalized agreements between the organizations. "In our kind of culture it is easy to reach an agreement on an informal basis, but we have to make sure that all of this is documented. The legal environment forces us to do things that aren't really natural for us."

*   Don't let the HMO get away from the clinic. A number of groups have allowed their HMO to drift apart from the clinic organization and then found themselves in an adversarial relationship with their primary source of revenue. While the monies made on an initial separation might be significant, the long-term negative relationships would not justify the funds received. We believe that owning, managing, and controlling our HMO has been a significant factor in making the overall Carle organization strong. Through our interorganizational agreements and negotiating relationship between the HMO and the hospital, we have also served that organization well by maintaining internal control.

*   Don't underestimate the reaction of competitors to strategic moves. We have seen cases where physicians and/or the hospital, in an effort to "close out Carle," have taken actions that, to us, do not appear reasonable to counter our presence.

*   Communicate, communicate, communicate with board members, physicians and other administrations. It is not possible to over communicate in an integrated organizational structure that has elements of suspicion just by virtue of the integrated, yet separate, organizations that we are.

*   Always assume there is another side to an issue. This is a factor that becomes more and more critical as organizations are integrated and the source of ideas become more dispersed. Allow your paradigms to shift.

- Significant issues don't always meet with initial acceptance, but it is critical in planning for the future of an integrated health care system that if the idea is good for the organization, it must be pursued time and time again until it is fully accepted. A number of issues from our history are good examples, namely the development of Family Practice, the development of our branch system and integrated HMO organization. All of these met with initial resistance, and it was only through strong leadership, principally Dr. Pollard, that we were able to accomplish these critical success strategies that have brought us to our present level of strength and positioned us well for health care reform.

Dr. Scully believes that to be successful in the future, an organization needs to be integrated across all variables that affect the delivery and cost of health care. "The most important are physicians, the hospital and the health plan. Long-term care, home health, rehabilitation, mental health and other services are also important. We need to think of it like a marriage."

Carle has learned that profitability is more important than market share, according to Dr. Scully. "We learned our lesson on this point in a couple of our HMO joint venture relationships. We couldn't control costs and this really impacted the profitability of our health plan as well as the clinic."

Issues for the Future

Kenneth Bash said that although Carle is a highly integrated system, there have been recent discussions about what to do next. "We are very concerned about the tightening of the application of fraud and abuse, and inurement laws. Although we have tried to be squeaky clean in the way we do business, we still feel vulnerable. If the feds want to encourage integrated systems, they are sending the wrong messages."

Carleton King said that he is concerned about the clinic's ability to shift over to a health care payment system totally based on capitation. "The physicians here work very hard, and they are rewarded on their productivity. Will we be willing to change the compensation system so physicians personally feel the responsibilities for the patients' health status?"

Dr. Scully was less worried about the ability of Carle to make the transition. "We can adjust our expenses and prices and control most of the variables that influence how we will do. We are about 50/50 primary care and this positions us well. Also this is a physician-owned and managed organization with a long history of working together."

King pointed out another dilemma for the future: "A significant number of referrals to Carle specialists still come from independent physicians in the region, and it would be unwise to do anything to discourage this source of business. At the same time, Carle has to be developing a system it can control, and this may be a closed system." Dr. Schrepfer had a different view: "I think people should act like professionals whether they are paid on a productivity basis or on a capitated basis. There are important ethical issues either way you go. I would hope we neither provide too little care, or too much."

Dr. Schrepfer also noted that one of the issues facing the clinic is whether to build more space or expand the hours and utilize the present space more effectively.

Board member Lykins said that Carle needs to strive for more complete integration. "In banking when we acquire a bank we can continue to keep the old management and operate as before. But, if we want to operate more efficiently and improve our financial performance, we have to integrate these acquired banks into our system. The same is true for the Foundation and clinic. There are two personnel offices and different wage and benefit policies. There are two housekeeping departments."

Dr. Pollard is worried about reimbursement in the future. "Will we have the financial resources to do what we need to do to be successful?" Dr. Parker said that he is concerned about eliminating administrative redundancies between the clinic and hospital and "changing specialists' and hospital management's mind set from generating revenues to being cost centers under a capitated payment system. This is a complete flip flop from what we are doing today."

NOTE: We thank Kenneth Bash and his staff for their assistance in scheduling the interviews and providing the background information used in preparing this case study.

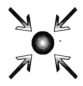

Case Study #5

SUTTER HEALTH
Sacramento, California

— Persons Interviewed —

Patrick Hays, President and CEO, Sutter Health
Gary Susnara, Senior Vice President,
    Health Systems Management, Sutter Health
Thomas Atkins, MD, Physician Manager,
    Sacramento Sierra Medical Group
Maurice Gloster, MD, Medical Director, Sutter Health
Van Johnson, President and CEO, Sutter Community Hospitals
Neil Pennington, member of the Sutter Health
    Board of Directors
Harold Ray, MD, member of the Sutter Health Board
    of Directors; President, Capitol Medical Group
Kurt Sligar, MD, Senior Vice President, Medical Affairs,
    Sutter Health
Dale Terry, Interim President, Sutter Preferred Health Plan

July, 1993

EXHIBIT A.
Sutter Health
Health Care Network

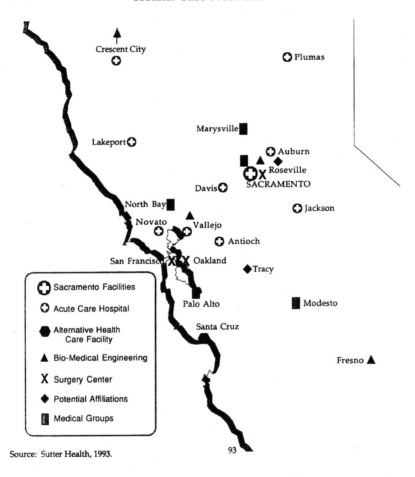

Crescent City

Plumas

Marysville

Lakeport

Auburn

Roseville

X

SACRAMENTO

Davis

Jackson

North Bay

Novato

Vallejo

Antioch

San Francisco X X Oakland

Tracy

Sacramento Facilities

Acute Care Hospital

Alternative Health Care Facility

Bio-Medical Engineering

X Surgery Center

Potential Affiliations

Medical Groups

Palo Alto

Modesto

Santa Cruz

Fresno ▲

93

Source: Sutter Health, 1993.

SUTTER HEALTH
Sacramento, California

This case study focuses on the development of Sutter Health as an integrated delivery system with special emphasis on the role of physicians in this process, especially the Sacramento Sierra Medical Group (Sac Sierra or SSMG).

Formed in late 1984, Sac Sierra was the first "clinic without walls" in the United States, and has been widely studied and emulated by physicians and other health care systems. In early 1992 the status of Sac Sierra changed, becoming the for-profit physician group providing services for the Sutter Medical Foundation, one of five such foundations formed within Sutter Health.

Based in Sacramento, Sutter Health operates facilities throughout Northern California.

The Sacramento Health Care Marketplace

The Sacramento Metropolitan Area is the fifth largest in California with a 1990 population of 1.5 million. Exhibit A shows the location of Sacramento and Sutter Health facilities throughout the northern portion of the state. Sacramento is the state capital, and its economic base is heavily dependent upon state and federal employment. It is also the center of a large and prosperous agricultural area, both the Central and San Joaquin Valleys.

The Sacramento health care market is dominated by managed care; Kaiser Permanente was the largest organization with 405,000 members in March, 1992. Foundation Health (FH), a for-profit organization, had 170,000 members in the area. Although there were a number of other managed care companies, none had a significant market share. Over 80 percent of the private health care market was served by managed care plans, primarily HMOs.

In early 1993 there were an estimated 200,000 Medi-Cal (the California Medicaid program) patients in the Sacramento region.

In addition to Sutter Health, major hospitals and hospital systems in the Sacramento area included Kaiser (two hospitals with 145 and 304 beds respectively), the University of California Davis Medical Center with 470 beds and Mercy Healthcare.

Mercy Healthcare, which was finalizing its merger with Methodist Hospital in the Spring, 1993, will have five hospitals with a total of more than 1,000 beds. Mercy also includes the Medical Clinic of Sacramento, an 82-physician group that joined with Mercy in 1990. Mercy was part of Catholic Healthcare West, a statewide network of 14 hospitals.

Sutter Health, 1983 to 1993

Over the past decade, Sutter Health made several strategic moves designed to position itself as an integrated health care system with hospitals, several medical groups, health plans, ambulatory centers of all types, nursing homes and other facilities and services covering large portions of Northern California.

In 1983, Sutter consisted of two hospitals, Sutter General (275 beds) and Sutter Memorial (353 beds), both located near the center of Sacramento. There were 900 physicians, mostly in solo practice and in small groups, on the combined medical staff of the two hospitals, and a large proportion of these doctors officed near the hospitals.

By 1993, Sutter Health had total revenues of over $1.8 billion, and more than 15,000 employees. It included 13 hospitals representing over 2,000 beds. With five medical foundations, Sutter included clinics, such as the Palo Alto Medical Foundation (140 physicians), Gould/Sutter in central California (over 100 physicians), the SSMG group in the Sutter Medical Foundation (140 physicians in the Sacramento area) and Marysville Medical Group north of Sacramento (45 physicians). In 1992, Sutter earned $43 million in excess revenues. Exhibit B is an income and expense statement for Sutter Health for 1990, 1991 and 1992.

As of year end 1992, Sutter Health had assets of $785 million and a fund balance of $370 million (see Exhibit B).

Patrick Hays, President and Chief Executive Officer (CEO), Sutter Health, suggests that Sutter's "Vision for the '90s" encompasses "four lanes along a common road:

- We will seek to solidify our position as the leading regional health system in Northern California.

- We will become the preeminent health care system in the greater Sacramento area.

- We will work to achieve that preeminence on the basis of quality, cost effectiveness, financial stability, local commitment and value added to the communities we serve.

EXHIBIT B.
Balance Sheet and Revenues and Expenses, Sutter Health, 1990-1992 (in millions)

Balance Sheet	1992	1991	1990
Property and Equipment	$353	$319	$297
Cash and marketable securities	238	235	164
Other assets	194	136	121
Total assets	$785	$690	$582
Long-term debt	$269	$243	$216
Other liabilities	146	117	93
Fund balance	370	330	273
Total liabilities	$785	$690	$582
Revenues and Expenses			
Net patient service revenues	$523	$465	$431
Other revenues	90	69	u
Total revenues	$613	$534	$489
Salaries and benefits	$317	$268	$236
Other expenses	253	213	200
Total expenses	570	481	436
Net income before extraordinary	43	53	53
Extraordinary charge on	6	---	---
Net income available for	$37	$53	$53
Major Investing Activities			
Capital expenditures	$67	$51	$30
Principal payments on long-term	5	4	21
Total	$72	$55	$51

Source: 1992 Annual Report, Sutter Health, April 1993.

- We will continue to implement fiscally sound health care diversification which adds demonstrable value to the system (Sutter Health, Annual Report, 1991)."

"Sutter Health's vision for the 1990's can be simply stated. Sutter Health will enter the twenty-first century as the preeminent Northern California regional health care delivery system comprised of a select series of local networks delivering care of a distinctly higher value supported by a committed diversification strategy and an aggressive willingness to be innovative" (*The Vision for the 1990's,* October 23, 1991).

The Growth of Sutter Health as an Integrated Delivery System

Patrick Hays, who came to Sutter in 1980, reported there were four major strategic planning periods followed by decision making and implementation leading to the development of Sutter Health as it stood in early 1993.

According to Hays, "In 1980, there was no common vision of the future. I am a strong believer in the importance of strategic planning for a large, complex organization, and this is one of the first things we launched." At that time Sutter consisted of two Sacramento hospitals and a combined medical staff. "We had a survival mentality. We were focused on our financial position and the fact that we were losing market share to Kaiser Permanente."

Harold Ray, MD, an obstetrician, President of Capitol Medical Group and member of the Sutter Health Board of Directors, referred to the vision of Sutter Health. "You can't be a two-hospital system with hospitals located in the downtown area of Sacramento. The future was not bright for Sutter if this was our vision for the future." As a result of the various strategic planning efforts throughout the 1980s, Dr. Ray said that Sutter Health decided to position itself to provide a continuum of care to the people of Northern California.

Several factors at work nationally and in California set the stage for the next big phase of planning (what Hays called the second iteration) that began in 1983. Dr. Paul Ellwood and Professor Alain Enthoven of Stanford University were talking about the growth of "SuperMeds," large for-profit hospital systems. California still had certificate of need (CON) and hospitals were highly regulated. Also, in 1981 California enacted its pro-competitive contracting for Medi-Cal. In 1984, Hospital Corporation of America (a for-profit corporation) purchased Wesley Hospital in Wichita, Kansas, a not-for-profit hospital, and this concerned many community-based, not-for-profit hospitals, including Sutter.

This second round of planning led to Sutter joining Voluntary Hospitals of America (VHA). "One of the things we decided was that Sutter didn't want to become part of a for-profit system; this was an important decision. If we were going to stay independent we needed to make some changes. Another one of the questions we grappled with in 1983-84 was whether or not we should be more geographically dispersed, and we decided we should be. Also, it was decided to reorganize and have corporate directors — the forerunner of Sutter Health."

Referring to the 1986-87 period, Hays said that during that time, Sutter Health went through its third major planning cycle. One of the questions considered was: "What can we do about health care costs? Our hospitals were becoming giant intensive care units (ICUs) and the acuity of our patients was increasing. There didn't seem to be much we could do about this shift and its impact on hospital costs, except to create ways to treat people which kept them out of our expensive hospitals." Another major issue was whether or not to develop a continuum of care (e.g., long-term care, home health); the decision was that Sutter needed to develop services for patients being discharged from its hospitals.

The most recent planning effort took place in the late 1980s. Hays said, "We saw the future evolution of health care systems, and recognized that the glue that would hold them together was a financing mechanism. The question was: should we be in financing? Our response was that we should. This set the stage for our investment in Foundation Health (FH), a publicly-traded HMO. This was probably the best financial decision we ever made (over $70 plus million profit), but our worst strategic decision, due to subsequent clashes in strategic versus tactical thinking. It delayed us in terms of making our move into financing through the development of managed care systems that we owned."

During this late 1980s planning period, the board, management and physician leaders also decided that Sutter should strive to become the preeminent health care provider in the region. Hays said, "We didn't want to continue to see ourselves as an alternative to Kaiser Permanente. This decision helped us focus on moving ahead of Kaiser and took our attention off Mercy. It also forced us into looking at how we were going to work with physicians."

EXHIBIT C.
General Organizing Concept

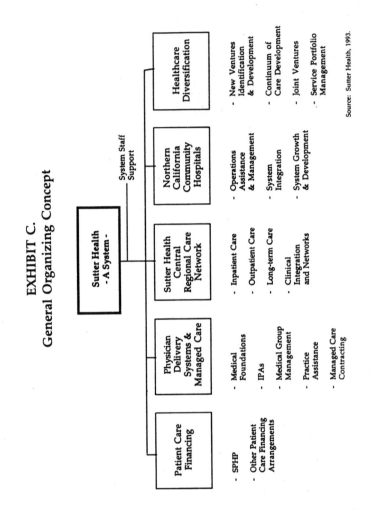

Source: Sutter Health, 1993.

Governance and Management of Sutter Health

Exhibit C is an organization chart for Sutter Health. The Sutter Health board consisted of seven individuals including one physician (Dr. Ray) and the President and CEO, Patrick Hays.

In the 1991 organizational realignment, services were clustered according to geography. For example, in Sacramento the Sutter Health Central Division included the three Sacramento acute care and psychiatric hospitals, plus two hospitals outside the metro area, skilled nursing, urgent care and home health. The remaining hospitals were gathered into another division known as Sutter Health Pacific.

Sutter Health's Approach to Physician Integration

Patrick Hays said that Sutter believes in a pluralistic approach to dealing with physicians. "Our physicians are wonderful human beings and they have supported us over the years. Our policy has been to offer them business-related assistance wherever we could. We never focused exclusively on Sac Sierra; we have offered a balanced program for all of our physicians." Neil Pennington, member of the Sutter Health Board of Directors and former Chairman, added that in 1990 Sutter Health made a decision to be pluralistic in its dealings with physicians; it would not turn its back on solo practitioners or small groups. He said that Sutter manages small group practices and supports IPAs across the geographic areas it serves.

The IPA. In 1982, the physicians at Sutter formed an IPA, called Capitol Medical Group. This was part of a decision to begin to think of physicians as functioning as part of the formal medical staff, but also having a need for a business relationship with one another. According to Kurt Sligar, MD, Senior Vice President, Medical Affairs, Sutter Health, "The entire medical staff was to continue to have responsibility for quality assurance and credentialing, but it would not have responsibility for business-oriented initiatives. You can't establish new business ventures with your leadership being elected for one or two year terms."

Dr. Sligar was the second president of Capitol Medical Group, and he was re-elected chairman in 1988. "My main objective during my second term was to get Sac Sierra and the IPA as exclusive providers for Foundation Health. After a long period of negotiations, we found out the president of FH never had any interest in such a proposal. He said, 'Do you think I am crazy? Why would I want to create an 800-pound gorilla?'"

Dr. Sligar said that in 1989, FH wanted to enter into a capitated relationship with Capitol Medical Group. "We went to the Sacramento Physician Network, the other major IPA in town and our major competitor, to see if they would like to join with us. They had experience in capitated contracts and we didn't. Also, although they were smaller, teaming up with them gave us a broader geographic base and this was appealing to health plans."

Dr. Ray, current president of the IPA, said that although Capitol Medical Group accepts capitated contracts, specialists are paid on a discounted fee-for-service basis with a 20 percent withhold. Primary care physicians, who are also paid on a discounted fee-for-service basis, have their performance evaluated every three months. Looking ahead, Dr. Ray said that the IPA may capitate a limited number of primary care physicians, perhaps 50.

There were 850 physicians in the IPA in April, 1993. Dr. Ray said the IPA was too large, with twice as many specialists as it needed. "This presents a difficult situation. If we tried to reduce the size of our physician panel, it would represent a severe economic blow to many specialists. On the positive side, people buying our IPA panel want as many physicians as possible so this makes it attractive from a marketing viewpoint."

Dr. Ray said that the IPA got into financial trouble in 1991 and Patrick Hays asked him to step in as president. "Sutter Health has put several million dollars into the IPA in the past couple of years, and it is now back on a sound financial footing."

In early 1993 the IPA had contracts with payors representing 68,000 lives. This compared with 24,000 patients covered by the Mercy IPA.

Practice support arrangements. Sutter Health, through its Physician Support Services Department, assisted 90 physicians in 1992. This department provides a wide range of contract support services, including marketing, strategic planning, office location and lease arrangement and overall practice management. The department supports local Sutter hospitals in recruiting new physicians to the community and helping them establish their practices.

Managed Care Systems became a wholly-owned affiliate of Sutter in 1992. This organization has assisted independent physician practices in negotiating and administering management care contracts and claims processing. This organization also functioned as a third-party administrator.

Relationships with additional medical groups. Sutter Health expanded its medical foundation model concept and its strategic objective of becoming an integrated system for Northern California, by forming new business arrangements with several clinics, including Palo Alto (140 physicians), Family Doctor Medical Group in Vallejo (30 physicians) and Gould Medical Foundation in Modesto (more than 100 physicians). Gould was the Central Valley's largest medical group and operated nine outpatient facilities throughout the region. More recently, Marysville Medical Group (now Sutter Medical Group-North) and its 40 physicians filled in the coverage gap north of Sacramento.

Maurice Gloster, MD, Medical Director, Sutter Health, summarized it in this way: "We have reaffirmed our commitment to plurality. But, within the medical community, there is no doubt about Sutter's commitment to the foundations."

Financing Mechanisms

As noted earlier, Sutter Health became an equity owner through a leveraged buy out of Foundation Health in 1986 and sold its interest three years later. It continued to be a provider for FH with this HMO representing less than 10 percent of the patients served by Sutter.

Sutter established Sutter Preferred Health Plan Services of Sacramento in 1985. Services included third-party administration. In June, 1992, Sutter Preferred purchased a 50 percent interest in Omni Health Plan, an HMO owned by VHA ally St. Joseph's Hospital in Stockton. The investment was $5 million.

When the interest in Omni Health Plan was purchased, the HMO had no members in the Sacramento area. Since that time, the HMO has increased its presence in Sacramento to 30,000 members in mid 1993.

Sacramento Sierra Medical Group (SSMG)

The Sacramento Sierra Medical Group, also known as Sac Sierra, was one of the best-known clinics without walls in the country. Over the past few years, several hundred physicians and hospital administrators have traveled to Sacramento to learn more about this organization.

SSMG was established in December, 1984, by 25 primary care physicians (mostly internists), an oncologist and two cardiologists. At the time it was absorbed into the Sutter Medical Foundation in early 1992, it had 147 physicians. Exhibit D shows the growth of the group, in terms of number of physicians, from its inception through 1992.

Origins of SSMG. Internist William Bush, MD, is often referred to as the key physician involved in the founding of SSMG. Regarding the formation of Sac Sierra, Dr. Bush said:

Nothing was being organized to bring physicians' medical training to bear on what the patient ought to have. And it also appeared that money was going to become the overriding factor. We felt that for physicians to have input in medical care, they were going to have to become a large corporate entity. Then they too could hire administrators to see that their input was at least listened to (*The Business Journal,* February 5, 1990).

According the Thomas Atkins, MD, Physician Manager for SSMG and a family practice physician who joined the group when it was six months old, the initial vision was that Sac Sierra would be a multispecialty clinic. "In addition," he added, "we also wanted to impact the health care environment rather than reacting to it. We wanted to be in a position to engage in direct contracting. And we wanted to have leverage at the bargaining table with payors, the hospital and others."

Robert Forster, MD, an internist and one of the SSMG founders, said, "We called it *our group practice without walls* — an experiment of sorts started in 1984 that combined centralized business operations with decentralized delivery of care." He went on, "It was a group made up of physicians with different interests, locations, hospital affiliations and specialties. The common vision was to organize an effective single business entity to maximize economic clout and yet preserve some traditional values of autonomy" (*The Internist,* October 1988, page 12).

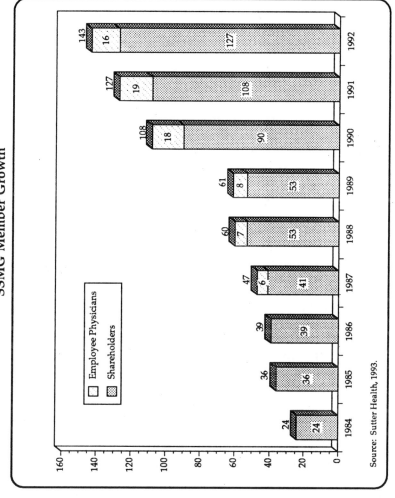

EXHIBIT D.
SSMG Member Growth

Source: Sutter Health, 1993.

Dr. Atkins said that specialists were not originally owners of SSMG. Specialists could purchase stock options which required them to pay Sac Sierra $400 per month. This allowed them to participate in the governance of the organization. Dr. Atkins also said, "We needed cash flow from the specialists to finance Sac Sierra. Early on we thought that primary care physicians could be financially viable, but this proved to be wrong. Kaiser Permanente bid up the price of primary care physicians in our area, and several members of our group began to look at the possibility of leaving for greener pastures. This put us in a difficult situation, and we needed money from specialists to maintain decent incomes for many primary care doctors."

Although the formation of SSMG was by physicians and independent of any hospital, Patrick Hays of Sutter said, "We were present at the birth of the Sac Sierra Medical Group. We said, 'What can we do to help?' My colleagues in the hospital administration field said we were crazy to encourage a group of physicians to organize and gain power." Hays pointed out, however, that the Medical Group of Sacramento had previously affiliated with Mercy, and no one paid much attention to it.

In looking back, Van Johnson, President and CEO, Sutter Community Hospitals, said, "The clinic without walls was really a subsidized IPA. It was like a chamber of commerce for small businesses. The physicians came together in response to a common vision, but they really did not come together from a cultural and operational point of view."

How Sac Sierra operated. Participating physicians were allowed to retain their offices (called care centers) and staff. In 1990, SSMG employed 65 people in its central office. The average monthly fee paid to the central office by participating physicians was $1,000, plus an additional amount based on a percentage of net revenues.

The central office also provided contracting assistance and pursuit of other business ventures, such as a clinical lab (later sold), cardiac diagnostic center, and a share of an endoscopy center. The central office provided services including purchasing, personnel, payroll and benefits, accounts payable, patient billing, malpractice insurance, contract administration, financial reporting and patient placement.

Sac Sierra was governed by a 12-member board of directors, with each director serving a three-year term.

Efforts to augment physicians' income. Looking back, Dr. Atkins said that in the 1984-85 period SSMG had the idea of owning an HMO. "We shopped and almost bought one. However, we changed our mind and saw contracting with a number of health plans as the way to go."

Dr. Atkins said that SSMG also established a laboratory, "But with the pressures from the Stark bill (legislation introduced by Congressman Pete Stark prohibiting physician self-referrals) and our concerns about fraud and abuse, we ended up selling it. In retrospect this was a bad decision because we lost an important source of ancillary income." He said that SSMG also bought an interest in an X-ray unit but did not own one by itself. The unit was co-owned with others and was profitable, but it did not represent a significant source of income for Sac Sierra. "One of our biggest mistakes was not to make sure we had a stream of ancillary income."

Dr. Atkins noted that SSMG was the preferred provider for many employers and individuals in Sacramento but was not delivering health care at the lowest cost. He noted that Kaiser did not accept Medi-Cal patients. Since many private practice physicians like those in Sac Sierra do serve Medi-Cal patients, this results in cost shifting for private sector physicians. "This is a significant amount of money and really hurt our competitive position with respect to Kaiser Permanente."

Dr. Atkins also described the money spent on information systems for SSMG. "We have burned through three information systems and are on our fourth. We are talking big bucks — on the order of $9 million. Physicians were supposed to be paying for this at the rate of $1,000 per month, but they aren't making the payments."

The financial crises of 1991. The legal and financial issues came to a head in February, 1991, and SSMG went into a strategic planning phase. Five months later, "Our vision was that we would become a multispecialty clinic, provide reasonable incomes for our members, and offer competitive costs for payors and patients. We estimated that we needed $20 million over five years to accomplish this."

Patrick Hays noted that in late 1991, "All hell broke loose for SSMG. We had to form the Sutter Medical Foundation, primarily because of concern over California's corporate practice of medicine laws and other potential legal issues. There were also financial issues, and SSMG needed an infusion of capital and operating revenues."

As a result of lower-than-expected physician incomes and other financial problems, SSMG's board began a search for a capital partner. (Several of the Sac Sierra internists were seriously thinking about leaving; their incomes were low compared with those offered by Kaiser Permanente.) According to Dr. Atkins, "We finally realized that we were horribly under-capitalized. To help this situation we began bringing in specialists; this distorted the composition and direction of the group."

Dr. Atkins went on to discuss the options for raising capital: borrowing (with personal guarantees of member physicians), capitalizing based on future earnings, and finding a financial partner. SSMG sent out a request for proposal (RFP) to such potential partners as Mercy, Sutter, PhyCor (a for-profit medical group management company) and Foundation Health (FH). Mercy backed out early. In the end, Sutter Health was the only organization that expressed substantial interest.

Atkins went on, "We — the board and members of SSMG — went through a terribly difficult decision-making process. At one meeting, which lasted over six hours, Sutter was approved as our financial partner by a six to five margin of our board. But no one felt good about it because of the perceived loss of control, and our members asked us to re-evaluate the alternatives. We did and came to the same conclusion — we had to have a capital partner and Sutter was our best bet. We went back to the members and everyone felt better. We decided to move ahead with Sutter."

The evolution into Sutter Medical Foundation (SMF). In May, 1992, Sutter Health completed the organization of Sutter Medical Foundation-Sacramento, the first medical foundation formed within Sutter Health. SMF's medical staff includes the physicians from Sac Sierra.

Robert Rowland, former administrator of SSMG, said that the organization decided to explore the foundation model when strategic planning revealed the need for growth in both the number of primary care physicians and geographic service area. "The planning process revealed that our top priorities would be access to capital to finance growth and to adequately compensate new primary care physicians. We looked at the alternatives and decided that the foundation model clearly made the most sense to our leadership" (*Physician Relations Advisor*, March 1992, page 46).

The Sutter Medical Foundation (SMF) was a non-profit corporation that owned and operated outpatient medical care facilities. The

Foundation employed most non-physician personnel, contracted with third-party payers, provided business, administrative and financial services, leased facilities, owned all assets and incurred liabilities. The Foundation compensated SSMG for medical services through a professional services agreement. Exhibit E shows the organizational chart for the foundation and Exhibit F shows the relationship of SMF to other Sutter Health entities. In mid-1993, 30 percent of SMF's revenues were derived from capitated managed care contracts.

SSMG remains a physician-owned, for-profit professional corporation. "While the Medical Group will not be initially linked to any other physician group, it is the intention and desire of SSMG, the Sutter Medical Foundation, and Sutter Health to ultimately merge two or more such physician organizations in northern and central California. The goal is to achieve greater economy and efficiency through the sharing of administrative functions and quality practices common to large medical groups" (Sutter Health, *A report, The Medical Foundation Model,* October, 1992).

Physicians who were members of SSMG were paid to provide care to the Sutter Medical Foundation's patients through a Professional Services Agreement. This agreement provided compensation for several aspects of service, including physician staff, physician benefits, quality assurance and utilization review, credentialing, and physician recruiting.

Gary Susnara, Senior Vice President, Health Systems Management, said that the Foundation would reduce the number of physicians from 140 to 100 with most of those dropping out being specialists. This would transform the Sutter Medical Foundation into a predominantly primary care group serving the Sacramento area. Van Johnson said, "The Sutter Medical Foundation has no business having specialists. Its primary purpose is to recruit and retain primary care physicians."

In the Sutter Medical Foundation/SSMG relationship, the physician compensation arrangement called for each primary care physician to receive $20,000 over and above what they generated from their productivity. Dr. Atkins said, "We proposed a $2 million per year salary supplement package, but this included the specialists. We finally settled for $1.2 million, which excludes specialists. Sutter said they could justify this amount."

EXHIBIT E.
Sutter Health Organizational Chart

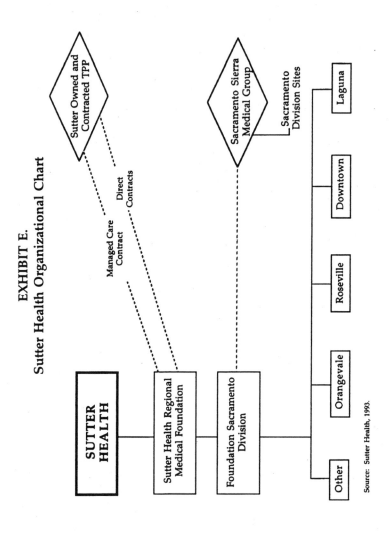

Source: Sutter Health, 1993.

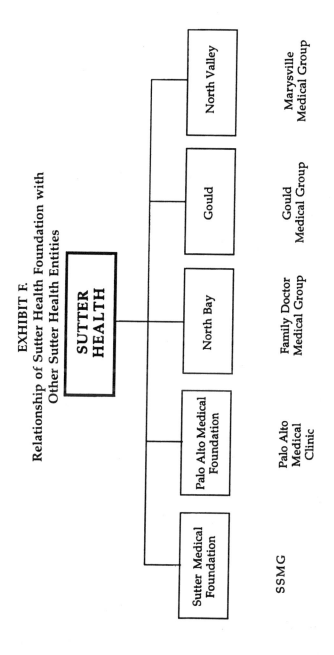

EXHIBIT F.
Relationship of Sutter Health Foundation with Other Sutter Health Entities

SUTTER HEALTH

Sutter Medical Foundation — SSMG

Palo Alto Medical Foundation — Palo Alto Medical Clinic

North Bay — Family Doctor Medical Group

Gould — Gould Medical Group

North Valley — Marysville Medical Group

Source: Sutter Health, 1993.

Gary Susnara said Sutter Health was fixing one of the problems of the "clinic without walls" model by moving toward building a limited number of medical plazas. (These plazas were a modification of the more ambitious concept of integrated medical campuses.) One medical plaza was opened in the south part of Sacramento in April, 1993, and two more were planned in areas where primary care physicians loyal to Sutter were needed. Susnara said, "As part of this we will consolidate most of the primary care sites (the 70 offices of physicians in SSMG) into a limited number of locations; this will be more cost effective and allow us to be more successful in generating ancillary income."

Primary Care Strategies

As noted above, Sutter completed construction of the Sutter Medical Plaza/Laguna (a suburban area in the southern part of Sacramento) in 1993, and broke ground for another plaza in Orangevale in the northeast area.

In 1992, two urgent care facilities were converted into community clinics. The clinics, located in south Sacramento and Rancho Cordova, made primary care services available to Medi-Cal patients.

Gary Susnara said that Sutter's primary care base in the Sacramento region was eroding. "Kaiser Permanente has had much more success in recruiting new primary care physicians than the rest of us. Nevertheless, we hope to add 15 to 20 primary care docs over the next year or so."

Neil Pennington added, "We decided in 1990 that primary care group practice was the name of the game. Sac Sierra was the only group that fit the bill." According to Pennington, the pressure point was Kaiser Permanente, and to be competitive, Sutter had to move into primary care more aggressively. Van Johnson agreed, "If you don't have a primary care base, you can't contract."

Other Aspects of Sutter Health

Total quality management (TQM). Sutter Health initiated TQM in 1989 and was well into the process. The focus has been on redesigning patient care and administrative procedures. Affiliated hospitals and physicians began TQM training during 1992. More than two dozen TQM projects had been completed by mid-1993.

Outcomes measurement/information systems. In discussing the importance of being able to measure outcomes, Dr. Sligar said, "This will give us a big advantage." He noted that Sutter was creating a common database. "No one around the country has such a system; everyone is doing it a little differently. There is no cookie cutter approach." He said that development of such a system will cost millions of dollars for the next few years, and that the board of Sutter Health is committed to such an expenditure.

In Sutter Health's 1992 *Annual Report*, the organization reported that, "Using Integrated Computer Aided Software Engineering technology, Sutter's system ultimately will pool medical records and cost information from its numerous affiliates. This database will allow the organization to review patient outcomes for efficiency and effectiveness, to enhance quality and help to contain or reduce costs in a resource-constrained era. Once in place, the computer link also will make Sutter more user-friendly to its patients since their medical records will follow them electronically into any Sutter facility they may use."

Gary Susnara said, "The piece we are struggling with is the information system. We are looking at millions of dollars to build this system, but we have to have it in order to manage the care of a large population. We will fail if we don't tie our system together with a sophisticated information system." (Richard Oszustowicz of Lifespan in Minneapolis and the University of Minnesota joined Sutter as Senior Vice President for System Integration to address the information management and telecommunications aspects.)

Other initiatives. Sutter was involved in a for-profit joint venture to build and operate outpatient surgery centers. At the end of 1992 the company, Sutter Surgery Centers, Inc., was involved with five owned and four managed surgery centers.

Lessons Learned — Clinic Without Walls

In looking back over the experience of SSMG, several individuals offered their perspectives on the experiment.

Dr. Atkins said, "The clinic without walls was a transitional model on the road to appropriate integration of provider systems to be able to respond to the market forces that exist." He also said that to be successful an organization has to focus on primary care. "We can't do this and also meet the needs of specialists. We told the specialists that we couldn't protect them from changes in the environment, but they wouldn't listen. They blamed us when they found they weren't doing as well as they expected."

Dr. Sligar characterized the lessons learned as follows:

(1) In looking back, the formation of SSMG was a necessary first step in an evolutionary process. If the physicians hadn't done it the way they did, with concern over autonomy and maintaining old practice styles, I don't think it would have been possible to get enough support to put a group together.

(2) The biggest mistake with SSMG was adding specialists. Furthermore, several of the specialists did not have cooperative attitudes and were not willing to make the necessary financial sacrifices to make the group work.

(3) You can't create a group democratically. The group has to learn to delegate to a board and a few leaders.

(4) You must have access to ancillary sources of income, such as laboratory and radiology, or the group won't survive. A primary care medical group needs a source of operating funds.

Dr. Sligar added that the matter of generating ancillary income to support primary care, including the former SSMG primary care doctors, remained an issue in 1993.

Gary Susnara said, "The concept of a clinic without walls is flawed. This kind of organizational structure doesn't generate enough revenues to cover its costs. With around 70 practice sites, plus a corporate office, it is inefficient. There was no reduction in the number of employees and there were no economies of scale. And, this kind of group doesn't generate ancillary revenues to help subsidize its operations. If you started a clinic without walls from scratch today, you would get creamed."

Patrick Hays noted that Sac Sierra was the necessary first step for the group, and that without this, it would not have been possible to form the Sutter Medical Foundation. (According to California law regarding the corporate practice of medicine, foundations have to have at least 40 physicians in order to become a foundation.)

---

* Gary Susnara and his staff arranged the interviews and pulled together the background information for this case study; we very much appreciated their help.

Case Study #6
UNIHEALTH AMERICA
Los Angeles, California

— Persons Interviewed —

Benjamin Snyder, Executive Vice President, UniMed America
Paul Alcala, Chief Information Officer, UniHealth America
H. Steven Ahoronian, MD, President, Facey Medical Group
Jeffrey Flocken, CEO, Northridge Hospital Medical Center
Reggie Friesen, MD, Huntington Provider Medical Group
John Harbourne, Executive Vice President, Bellflower Medical Group
Howard LeVant, Executive Vice President, UniHealth America and
    Coordinator, Long Beach ODS
Michael Lynch, MD, Facey Medical Group
Robert Nelson, Executive Vice President, Harriman-Jones Medical Group,
    Long Beach
Robbe Rygg, Chief Financial Officer, UniHealth America Ventures
Dennis Strum, Senior Vice President for Corporate Development,
    UniHealth America

July, 1993

EXHIBIT A.
Locations of UniHealth America Hospitals and Medical Groups

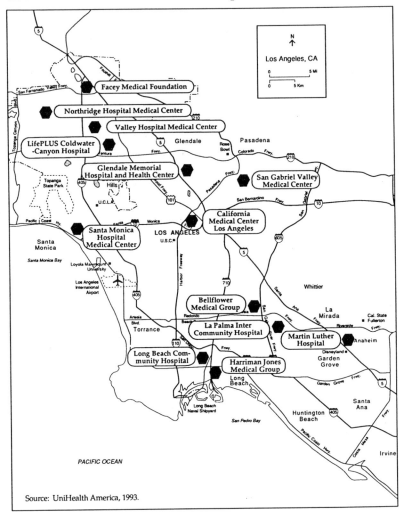

Source: UniHealth America, 1993.

UNIHEALTH AMERICA
Los Angeles, California

UniHealth America's vision is to manage the health of defined populations in known markets. Created in 1988 through the merger of two nonprofit organizations — HealthWest Foundation and LHS Corporation — the system provides the framework for an array of affiliated health care resources. By the end of 1992, UniHealth consisted of two large health maintenance organizations (HMOs), 4,300 physicians on the medical staffs of 11 acute care hospitals and a host of health-related businesses. The consolidated net revenues of UniHealth, for the fiscal year ending September 30, 1992, were more than $3.2 billion, of which two thirds were from managed care (capitated) contracts. UniHealth was one of the nation's five largest voluntary nonprofit health care networks.

Ben Snyder, Executive Vice President, UniMed America (the physician-oriented component of UniHealth), said, "Our objective has shifted away from being a hospital company to being an integrated health care system directed toward provider networks and long term relationships with major payors/health plans. Only 35 percent of our company's revenues now come from inpatient care."

UniHealth America is located in the competitive Los Angeles health care market, where managed care (defined as capitated systems) is predominant. Exhibit A shows the location of UniHealth and its affiliates.

The Los Angeles Health Care Marketplace

Growth in managed care. With its 15 million residents, the Los Angeles area is one of the most heavily populated managed care markets in the United States. Kaiser Permanente, the largest health care system in the area, had over two million subscribers in 1993.

Major health plans, mostly capitated, operating in early 1993 were:

Name of Plan	No. of Subscribers
(1) Kaiser	2,250,000
(2) HealthNet	1,000,000
(3) PacifiCare	200,000
(4) TakeCare	150,000
(5) Foundation Health	300,000

The largest medical groups. The Permanente Medical Group was the largest in the Los Angeles area with 3,200 physicians; Permanente hired 1,000 new physicians during the 1980s. Kaiser Permanente operated 93 sites in the area.

The Mullikin Medical Centers, a medical group practice started by Walter Mullikin, MD, in 1956, had 400 physicians (two thirds in primary care) and 287,000 managed care enrollees. Mergers during the past 12 months added seven medical groups with over 200 physicians. According to Dr. Mullikin, 80 percent of the clinic's business is capitated (*AMA News*, April 12, 1993). The group also owned 99-bed Pioneer Hospital in Artesia.

Pacific Physician Services (PPS) was a 140-physician group started by Gary Groves, MD. Groves took the company public in 1991 and raised $17.3 million. Loma Linda University Medical Center owned seven percent of PPS. PPS had 150,000 covered lives in 15 capitated agreements and operated 23 sites.

Friendly Hills HealthCare Foundation in La Habra had 150 salaried physicians in 10 sites and had 100,000 enrollees in 18 HMO contracts. It received Internal Revenue Service approval for tax-exempt status in early 1993. The organization also owned a 163-bed hospital, the Friendly Hills Regional Medical Center.

California Primary Physicians, a for-profit group located in downtown Los Angeles, had 150 salaried physicians at 20 sites. It had 125,000 enrollees under 10 managed care contracts.

Hospitals. The Los Angeles area had 210 hospitals with 45,000 licensed beds in 1992. Thirty hospitals had closed since 1981. The average utilization rate was 63 percent.

History of UniHealth America and Development as an Integrated Delivery System

Early history. In 1975, the hospital components of what is now UniHealth were Northridge Hospital Medical Center in the San Fernando Valley and California Medical Center, Los Angeles. Each would become the nucleus of two separate health care organizations, HealthWest Foundation and LHS Corporation, respectively.

A number of significant factors led to the formation of multihospital systems, in particular, California's certificate of need (CON) laws made it nearly impossible for hospitals, operating near capacity, to add beds. Northridge addressed the problem through the purchase of a nearby hospital in Van Nuys. Similarly, LHS Corporation expanded to include additional acute care facilities. The impetus for the formation of HealthWest Foundation, in 1979, was provided by Northridge's growth. By 1988, HealthWest was composed primarily of nine hospitals and Care America Health Plan, while LHS Corporation consisted of three acute care facilities and PacifiCare Health Systems, Inc.

The merger leading to the creation of UniHealth America. The merger between HealthWest Foundation and LHS Corporation occurred in June, 1988. Samuel Tibbitts, former president of LHS and later Chairman of the Board of UniHealth America, described the merger as "a once in a lifetime opportunity to increase market share and create a dramatically superior network. More importantly, the two nonprofit organizations share a common vision of providing the best possible care to our patients at a reasonable cost. This merger allows us to continue to fulfill that mission in an increasingly competitive health care arena" (from the charter issue of *Envisage*).

UniHealth America in early 1993. Exhibit B shows UniHealth's major operating groups. UniHealth America Ventures is the for-profit arm of the non-profit UniHealth America system.

As noted, UniHealth America operated 11 acute care hospitals ranging in capacity from 200 to 444 beds. The locations of these hospitals are shown in Exhibit A. Along with the Los Angeles area hospitals, UniHealth owned 200-bed Meadowlands Hospital in New Jersey.

By 1993, UniHealth had two HMOs and a preferred provider organization (PPO) network: CareAmerica (250,000 subscribers),

EXHIBIT B.
UniHealth Management Organization

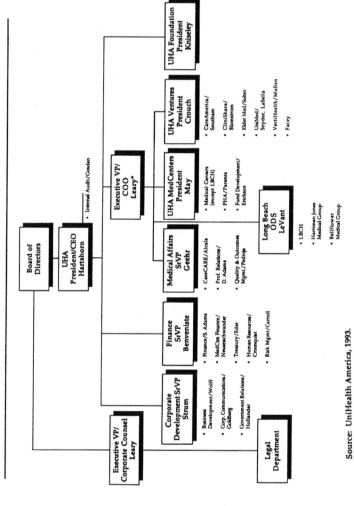

Source: UniHealth America, 1993.

publicly-traded PacifiCare (more than one million members in five states) and the PPO Alliance (700,000 members in California). UniHealth owned a majority interest in Class A voting shares of PacifiCare. Along with the revenue from its own managed care organizations, UniHealth realized two-thirds of its 1992 total revenues by servicing subscribers of several dozen managed care plans, nearly all of which required risk contracting.

Other divisions of UniHealth included CliniShare, ElderMed America and VertiHealth. The CliniShare division provided pre- and post-hospital services (e.g., home health, hospice care, respiratory therapy, and medical equipment). ElderMed focused on the development of a comprehensive range of services designed to preserve the integrity, individuality, and wellness of over 500,000 seniors nationwide. VertiHealth complemented the other divisions by acting as the network's contracting arm; this division synthesized relationships with numerous health plans, self-insured employers and brokers.

UniMed America. UniMed was formed to assist physicians in developing, building and managing their practices. This division of UniHealth was the vehicle for a group of services that included physician recruitment, practice enhancement consulting, IPA management, management information systems (including computer communication networks for physicians and hospitals) and management through services to foundations and organizations.

Recent changes in strategic direction. In the spring of 1993, the UniHealth America board of directors approved a series of "refinements" to the company's vision and strategic direction. These were designed to clarify the steps necessary for transition from a multihospital system to a network of Organized Delivery Systems (ODS).

The ODS concept, as defined by UniHealth, describes a network of organizations that provides, or arranges to provide, a coordinated range of services (physicians, hospitals, after-care) to a defined population and is willing to be held clinically and fiscally accountable for the health of the population served. The concept of an ODS is presented graphically in Exhibit C.

The initial ODS included Long Beach in early 1993. The San Fernando Valley and the greater San Gabriel Valley were also targeted for potential ODS development. Dennis Strum, Senior Vice President for Corporate Development, UniHealth America, said the result will be that UniHealth will be more tightly focused geographically, ensuring a better understanding of its customers' needs.

EXHIBIT C.
UniHealth America's Organized Delivery System

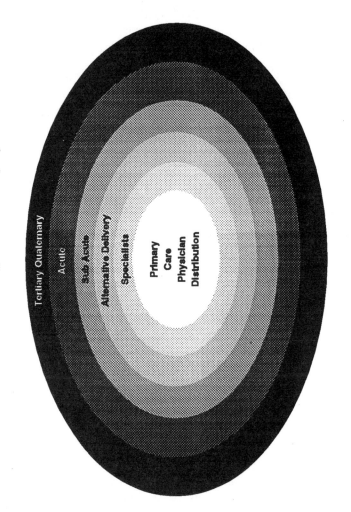

Tertiary Quaternary

Acute

Sub Acute

Alternative Delivery

Specialists

Primary
Care
Physician
Distribution

Source: UniHealth America, 1993.

Strum continued, "Our new strategy will entail an evolutionary process with the goal of achieving multiple local market-dominant positions. We will then link these markets together to compete regionally." This concept is illustrated in Exhibit D.

"In essence, we're transitioning from a hospital-based system to a health care system with the physician at the core of everything we do," said Strum. The new paradigm represented by this shift is illustrated in Exhibit E. "For example, we are moving from being asset based to being relationship based, and from hospital centered to physician centered. Instead of seeing ourselves as managers of episodes of care, we want to manage the health status of a defined population. Rather than pursuing strategies that are in the best interest of the institution, we are looking at the best interest of the customer."

The next three sections focus on recent developments in three of the proposed UniHealth ODS sites — Long Beach, San Fernando Valley and northern Orange County.

Harriman Jones Medical Group/Long Beach Community Hospital

The Long Beach ODS included the newly affiliated Harriman Jones Medical Group and Long Beach Community Hospital (329 beds). The service area encompassed an eight-mile radius containing close to one million persons; Harriman Jones served approximately 10 percent of the market. The medical group had three other locations within the service area.

Harriman Jones was in direct competition with the Mullikin Medical Group, headquartered only 15 miles away, as well as with several other relatively large medical groups located approximately the same distance from Long Beach, such as CIGNA and Kaiser. Kaiser Permanente had approximately 20 percent market penetration in the Long Beach area.

Established by Harriman Jones, MD, in the 1930s, the group had 80 full-time equivalent physicians, including 32 to 35 primary care doctors, in early 1993. According to Robert Nelson, Executive Vice President, "We see 1,100 patients a day and we have 46,000 managed care subscribers, plus another 5,000 in a senior HMO. These two sources represent 90 percent of our practice."

EXHIBIT D.

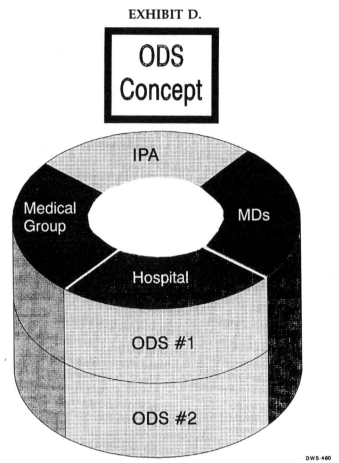

Source: UniHealth America, 1993.

EXHIBIT E.

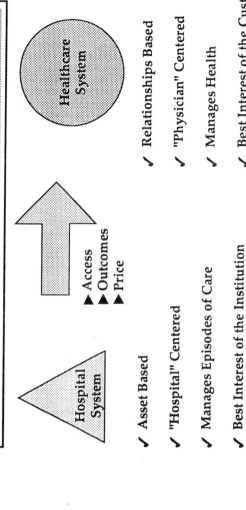

A Systematic Change Process

Hospital System

Healthcare System

▲ Access
▲ Outcomes
▲ Price

✓ Asset Based
✓ "Hospital" Centered
✓ Manages Episodes of Care
✓ Best Interest of the Institution
✓ Institutional Based Planning

✓ Relationships Based
✓ "Physician" Centered
✓ Manages Health
✓ Best Interest of the Customer
✓ Market Based Planning

Source: UniHealth America, 1993.

The group signed its first HMO contract in 1975. Nelson said, "In the 1982 through 1987 period, HMO enrollment in the Long Beach area exploded. We were growing at 15 to 30 percent each year just to keep up."

He went on, "In a capitated environment we know that primary care is the engine. When we look at specialists, we look at them as dollars spent in order to provide care for our subscribers. Whether or not we add specialists is really a 'make or buy' decision."

The leaders of the Harriman Jones Medical Group began talking to UniHealth America in 1990. Nelson said:

> We represented about one-third of the admissions to Long Beach Community Hospital, which was part of UniHealth. Given the volatility of the Los Angeles market, hospital management was concerned that we might join with another group. From our perspective, we were seeing the market change. It was going to take capital to continue to compete. For example, it costs about a half a million dollars to establish a satellite office, and we needed more of them. We saw UniHealth as a strong system, a survivor. We started talking.

The negotiations began in May 1991 and the deal was made effective January 1, 1992. A decision was made to apply for foundation status and approval was pending in April, 1993.

Howard LeVant, Executive Vice President, UniHealth America and Coordinator, Long Beach ODS, said that UniHealth and the Long Beach Community Hospital will be working to establish an IPA in the area. "This is part of our philosophy of working with physicians in all types of practice situations. We aren't turning our backs on anyone."

LeVant, a former administrator of the Long Beach Community Hospital, noted that the hospital's occupancy rate was averaging 180 inpatients, about double the utilization five years earlier, and it was profitable. "The hospital is really geared up for managed care and is very low-cost and efficient."

In looking back, Nelson said that leaders of the medical group and management of Long Beach Community Hospital had been meeting for one to two hours every Thursday morning for six years. This helped develop a mutual respect and rapport between physicians and hospital executives and set the stage for the development of the new medical foundation. Nelson said, "In looking back, the physicians feel that they made the right decision."

Nelson continued, "Looking ahead, our vision is to become the dominant provider in the Long Beach area. This will mean increasing our market share to about 20 percent. We have a business plan designed to get us where we want to go."

Facey Medical Group/Northridge Hospital

Facey Medical Center and Northridge Hospital Medical Center were two of the key components of the proposed San Fernando Valley ODS.

The Facey Medical Group was established in 1923. It had grown to 76 full-time equivalent physicians in mid-1993. Facey was a multispecialty clinic with an internal medicine/pediatrics base. It covered 48,000 lives; this compared with 20,000 lives five years earlier. It operated four satellites (including one adjacent to Northridge Hospital) plus its home office. Facey received Internal Revenue Service approval for foundation status in late March, 1993. Facey Medical Foundation contracts with Facey Medical Group to be its exclusive physician provider.

The payor mix of the Facey Medical Group was 75 to 80 percent managed care (capitated), 12 percent Medicare and Medi-Cal, with the rest private pay or indemnity.

Gastroenterologist H. Steven Ahoronian, MD, President of Facey Medical Group, said, "Managed care changed the structure of the group. It made us more dependent on primary care. This changed our outlook. Now we try to figure out how many specialists we need and compare the cost of hiring someone, with going outside for these services."

Dr. Ahoronian said that to reach the critical mass needed to be successful in managed care (probably around 60,000 lives), "we needed a partner. We prepared a business plan; we were very deliberate about this. We could see that we needed $5 to $7 million over the next five years for a new main building, computer systems and imaging equipment. We looked at two or three potential partners, mostly hospital systems. We wanted a partner that was vertically integrated and UniHealth looked good. Plus, they were a local player."

On the question of loss of autonomy by virtue of the relationship with UniHealth, Dr. Ahoronian answered, "I am not sure we lost our autonomy; managed care imprisoned us several years ago."

Looking ahead Dr. Ahoronian said, "It is conceivable that we could double our size. To do this we are going to have to continue to build our primary care base."

Along with the Facey Medical Group, the 427-bed Northridge Hospital Medical Center was also part of the proposed San Fernando Valley ODS. Jeff Flocken, CEO of Northridge Hospital Medical Center, said, "Over the last 12 to 18 months we have had a 13 percent reduction in average length of stay. However, this killed us financially since we still have fee-for-service business. It probably cost us $6 million in lost profits. It is hard to have our feet in two different worlds, but we are committed to much more aggressive case management to keep our costs down."

Northridge has become a pluralistic organization, doing business with IPAs, medical groups and other physician practices. Flocken said the hospital had a medical staff of 750, with 220 being active and admitting most of their patients to Northridge. A local IPA had 27 primary care physicians and 75 to 100 specialists and was responsible for 48,000 enrollees in eight or nine risk contracts. "We work closely with the IPA on these contracts. We have a joint operations committee that meets every two weeks to review problem patients, system problems and contract performance. The IPA has a full-time medical director and we all work hard to control inpatient utilization."

In addition, there was another physician group that provided a panel for non-capitated contracts (e.g., preferred provider organizations -- PPOs). Almost all of the physicians associated with the hospital were part of this group, and it had over 100 contracts. Flocken said, "We will also work with this group as long as the market provides these kinds of products. However, these PPOs are beginning to look more and more like HMOs."

In another example of how the hospital worked with physicians, Flocken said that in 1990 a nine-member primary care group located near the hospital was having management and financial problems. He helped facilitate a merger of this medical group with the Facey Medical Foundation. "This was good for all concerned."

Flocken pointed out that the Mullikin Medical Clinic operated a site adjacent to the hospital, and it was staffed with 12 or 13 physicians. The Northridge group of Mullikin had the responsibility for 30,000 lives. "We are their primary hospital."

In summary, Flocken said that Northridge was not a low-cost hospital, largely because of several tertiary care services (e.g., neonatal intensive care and cardiovascular surgery). "It is going to take a lot of new relationships to keep this asset working. Our role is different and difficult; we have to manage through the transition. Our goal is to capture 20 percent of the market. If we can't reach this goal, we can't be assured of being a significant player in the marketplace."

Kaiser Permanente had two hospitals in the area and had 12 percent of the market. Flocken added, "There are 20 hospitals in the Valley and we probably only need one quarter or one third of these."

Bellflower Medical Group

Located in the northern part of Orange County, the Bellflower Medical Group had 14 physicians, 13 in primary care and one surgeon. It had two locations in 1993, including one adjacent to the La Palma Intercommunity Hospital, a UniHealth facility. The Bellflower Medical Group was the largest admitter of patients to this 136-bed hospital.

The group had 14,500 lives covered in capitated contracts in early 1993. According to John Harbourne, Executive Vice President, Bellflower Medical Group, the number of lives covered was down from 16,500 two years earlier. "This area has been particularly hard hit by layoffs in the aerospace industry, and this has impacted our group. One of our major accomplishments has been to adjust to this decline."

In 1992, UniHealth affiliated with the Bellflower Medical Group and agreed to provide administrative support to the clinic through a management services organization (MSO). As a part of this agreement, the medical group would receive a negotiated fixed percentage of net revenues for the last two years. In return, the group signed a 20-year management agreement with UniHealth America.

Harbourne said that the primary factors motivating the owners of Bellflower Medical Group to enter into a relationship with UniHealth were being able to access the capital structure of a larger organization and the likelihood that UniHealth would be one of the surviving organizations in the marketplace.

The professional corporation, Bellflower Medical Group, had four shareholders. However, ownership was to be expanded to all physicians, including nine primary care physicians who were in solo practice in the area, but who would be joining the group before the end of 1993. "For these physicians, who have predominantly fee-for-service (Medicare, PPOs) patients, a primary motivating factor for joining is to gain access to managed care contracts and to achieve economic stability." Harbourne noted that these physicians were making more money than those in the Bellflower Group, but that the higher level of earnings could not be maintained given the continuing trend toward managed care.

Harbourne explained that new primary care physicians were brought into the group at salaries of $100,000, and that earnings usually increase to around $120,000 within four or five years. When asked about incentives for productivity, Harbourne said, "There usually isn't much left to distribute, but we do reward physicians for various activities they are involved with. Being 90 percent managed care, I tell our physicians that when they come to work and the parking lot is empty they are making money; when it is full they are probably losing money."

Looking ahead, Bellflower Medical Group considered itself to be a key element in the ODS planned for northern Orange County. Affiliations with two area hospitals, La Palma Intercommunity Hospital and Martin Luther Hospital, both UniHealth facilities, are foreseeable. This may mean eventual expansion to the point when the group will be large enough to qualify for a change to foundation status; this requires 27 full-time equivalent physicians in California.

Harbourne said that one of the "lessons learned" in operating a primary care practice in a capitated environment was the importance of the medical director. "This individual calls the shots on referring patients outside the system and on other key factors that affect patient care and our ability to be successful." He added, "In this health care environment you have to focus on today and tomorrow; you can't rest on your laurels."

All three of the groups — Harriman Jones, Facey and Bellflower — operated immediate care clinics that provided 24-hour service for their subscribers.

Other Aspects of UniHealth

Matrix management teams. The implementation of matrix management teams has been fundamental to UniHealth's post-merger achievements. These teams have been the vehicle by which change has been affected throughout the organization. In many instances , physicians have lead the teams and have fostered the blending of physician services with home health and health plan services.

Since the merger, UniHealth has used the team approach to differentiate itself from competitors in areas as diverse as emergency services, accounts receivable, clinical protocols, case management, and managed care.

Outcomes measurement. UniHealth has taken a broader approach to measuring outcomes, encompassing not only hospital outcomes, but also the physician piece. The view held by the organization is that "physicians are what sells and what drives the system," according to Dennis Strum.

Robbe Rygg, Vice President and Chief Financial Officer, UniHealth America Ventures, expands on this concept, "Hospitals deal with episodic care. As we integrate we will want data on both episodic care and encounters in physicians' offices. Our ultimate goal is to keep our population healthy, but when they do need our services we have to be able to prove that we are doing an excellent job and achieving top notch results."

Total quality management. UniHealth has an ambitious program called QUEST (Quality Utilizing Excellence, Service and Teamwork). In 1990, QUEST was formally adopted by all the network's operating units (CareAmerica, CliniShare, ElderMed, and the hospitals affiliated with UniHealth America). Teams at one of the hospitals have been involved in the following projects: patient billing, pre-operative patient education, emergency services wait time, patient internal transportation, employee back safety, pre-surgical admission process, and rehabilitation patient scheduling. Clinical teams at this hospital are involved in projects concerned with oxygen tank utilization, coordinating medical supplies equipment at discharge, antibiotic utilization, and DRG 89 (simple pneumonia).

Information system development. UniHealth has shifted its emphasis from traditional "legacy" applications, mainly focused around its hospital business activities, to a much broader view of the mission of information technology. According to Paul Alcala, Chief Information Officer, UniHealth America, "our job used to be simply to buy good systems at good prices and to be cost-effective in operating them. Now we have to create solutions to business problems that have never been solved before." In addition, the new business direction of the company requires it to work intimately with a host of organizations that were clearly separate, or even competitors, in the East. "This is a whole new area of technology for us, but one which offers exceptional returns in productivity," Alcala added.

UniHealth has aggressively pursued the development of health care communication systems as part of its integration strategy. Considerable resources have been invested in the creation of MedComm (Medical Communications Networks, Inc.). This system provides rapid, accurate and inexpensive communication of clinic data among health care providers.   Although focused on physicians, the network includes hospitals, clinical laboratories, diagnostic centers and other health care-related organizations.

UniHealth also has been an innovator in the automation of its managed care business activities. A comprehensive administrative system, MC400, first developed for its wholly owned HMO, CareAmerica, is now used in some form by all the divisions within UniHealth doing managed care business: medical groups, IPAs and hospitals. This system also is marketed nationally and was recently installed as the managed care system for Friendly Hills Medical Group and the Carle Clinic, among others.

To manage this diverse environment and to provide the foundation for outcomes measurement, UniHealth has also embarked on the development of an Enterprise Management System. This is a repository for data from every division within the system and will be accessible throughout the organization. According to Dennis Strum, an integrated view of the entire organization is essential. Each part of the organization is dealing with the same patients, and it is no longer possible to operate each business unit in isolation and remain competitive.

Strum noted that information systems in a capitated system need to provide "real time" information so changes can be made quickly. He said it is important to be able to constantly compare actual utilization against that projected from actuarial data (similar to budgeted versus actual financial data that executives of most organizations rely on to manage those organizations).

He also noted that information is very important in dealing with physicians. "They respond much better to data than to anecdotes."

Robbe Rygg discussed the need to build an "electronic data interchange." He said this kind of system would include the ability to process claims, prepare reports on patient encounters, determine eligibility (which patients are eligible for which services such as co-payments, deductibles), and a unified medical record. "In addition we want to integrate records for physicians and hospitals."

Corporate culture. No case study of UniHealth America would be complete without a description of several aspects of its culture. UniHealth faced a serious challenge of integrating two large organizations following the 1988 merger between LHS Corporation and HealthWest Foundation. One attempt at addressing this issue was the extensive use of matrix management teams (discussed earlier). Each team has 10 or 12 people working at all levels of the new organization.

Team UniHealth is another example of the efforts to speed along the development of a corporate culture. Each employee receives a 37-page playbook which introduces Team UniHealth as the people-to-people mobilization campaign.

Team UniHealth rallies involved 250 senior managers from throughout the network's hospitals, divisions, subsidiaries and corporate offices. During the first 100 days of UniHealth America, these celebrations were held frequently and have since assumed a three-times yearly schedule. One medical group manager new to UniHealth America said that he attended these rallies, and although the idea sounded "hokey," he enjoyed the time and thought it was productive.

The Team UniHealth program also includes a unifying anthem, the UniHealth Americans Chorus and the creation of the UniStore (T-shirts, coffee mugs, etc.). The 1992 <u>Annual Report</u> discussed the recognition of system "champions." UniHealth employees also had the opportunity to become involved in a program of community assistance called "Heal L.A." following the 1992 civil unrest.

Major Accomplishments

Considering its genesis from two hospital-based organizations located in the San Fernando Valley and downtown Los Angeles, UniHealth America has dramatically expanded its market share in the Los Angeles area. In the course, it has transformed itself from being a multihospital corporation, to an integrated health care system, encompassing the delivery and financing of regional health care.

There is little doubt but that UniHealth has learned how to be successful in a managed care environment. The organization knows how to market capitated contracts, and it is gaining experience in utilization management and the other techniques important to profitably managing the health of a defined population.

One of UniHealth's major accomplishments has been its ability to position itself for health care reform. Given the system's coverage of the Los Angeles area, it is well situated to be a surviving Accountable Health Partnership (AHP). UniHealth is refining its integration mission to include the goal of becoming the leading managed care organization in California. This effort is centered on primary care physicians and will involve the strategic deployment of capital resources that is closely correlated with market opportunities. To this end, meeting market needs is the primary focus of the new organization. The further pursuit of operational integration through the ODS concept will provide the framework for an organization that is sensitive to the market and political environments and will secure the creation of a strong state-wide system.

Lessons Learned

UniHealth's strategic focus on Organized Delivery Systems in four or five sub-areas within the greater Los Angeles area is one lesson learned. As one manager said, "We were definitely spread too thin. This market is so large it is almost impossible for one organization, even Kaiser Permanente, to be dominant throughout the Los Angeles area. We have learned to pick our targets; to deploy our assets more effectively."

UniHealth has learned that it must have programs for physicians in a wide variety of practice settings ranging from solo practice to small groups to larger groups. This has led to the development of practice support, formation and management of IPAs, creation of an MSO (Bellflower) and the formation of medical foundations (Harriman Jones and Facey).

Strum said that primary care physicians are in the position of power. "Doctors don't trade referrals in the lounge any more; it is based on quality and cost effectiveness." He added, "Physicians drive everything; they are the most critical stakeholders in a capitated system. We recognized this fact several years ago, but the reality is driven home with each passing day."

"We see two models emerging," said Strum. "On one side there will be the organized delivery systems with financial components like Kaiser Permanente. On the other side we see nonintegrated providers. They will be vendors or 'hospitals and specialists for rent.' The risks associated with just being a vendor are high. UniHealth does not want to be a vendor, we want to be in the first category."

Issues for the Future

Dennis Strum summarized his concerns about the future as:

(1) Availability of primary care physicians; they drive a capitated system and they are going to continue to be in short supply. Competition for those who are available will become more severe.

(2) Continued earnings and access to capital.

(3) Capitalizing on the brief window of opportunity. He is concerned that health care reform may come quickly and the time to prepare is limited.

(4) Managing the transition to a new health care system. This relates especially to hospitals that depend on Medicare and limited amounts of fee-for-service business while at the same time making the transition to being cost-effective for managed care contracting.

(5) Governance and financial accountability for the Organized Delivery Systems (ODS); this will require some new thinking.

(6) Doing a better job of managing the revenue (premium) stream.

In summary, Strum said, "There are many risks associated with what we are trying to do, but many potential benefits when we pull it off."

---

*Benjamin Snyder, Executive Vice President, UniMed America, and Keith McWilliams, Administrative Resident, UniMed America, coordinated the interviews and data collection associated with this case study; we appreciate their help.

Case Study #7

OREGON MEDICAL GROUP/
SACRED HEART HEALTH SYSTEM*
Eugene, Oregon

— Persons Interviewed —

Virginia Slate, Assistant Administrator, Sacred Heart Hospital
    and Chairperson, Oregon Medical Services Organization
James Schwering, Executive Director,
    Oregon Medical Services Organization
Wayne Atwood, member of the board, Sacred Heart Health System
    and Oregon Medical Services Organization
Loren Barlow, MD, founder, Oregon Medical Group
Robert Crist, MD, founder, Oregon Medical Group
Wesley Jacobs, MD, Vice President of Medical Affairs,
    Sacred Heart Health System
Mark Litchman, MD, past medical director, SelectCare

July, 1993

EXHIBIT A.

Location of Oregon Medical Center and Sacred Heart Health System

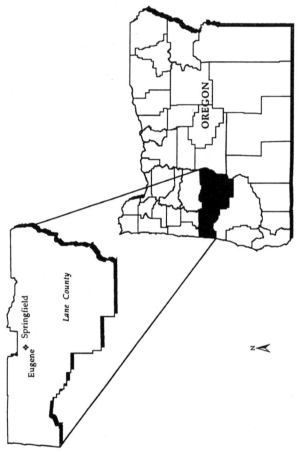

OREGON MEDICAL GROUP/
SACRED HEART HEALTH SYSTEM*
Eugene, Oregon

The Oregon Medical Group (OMG) was formed by 24 physicians in late 1988. By early 1993, the group included 53 primary care physicians operating out of seven locations in Eugene. The group had selected a management services organization (MSO) model.

Health and Hospital Services, a Catholic organization that owns Sacred Heart Hospital, a 450-bed tertiary care facility, has made a strong commitment to the integration of physicians, its health plan and the hospital. It has several other initiatives, in addition to OMG, for accomplishing this strategic objective.

The Eugene Health Care Marketplace

The community. In 1991, Lane County had a population of 290,000. Eugene, Oregon's second largest city, had 117,000 residents and is the home of the University of Oregon, which had an enrollment of 17,800 students. Springfield, just across the Williamette River and three miles from Eugene, had 45,000 residents. Exhibit A shows the locations of Eugene, Springfield and Lane County within the State of Oregon.

The economy of the area was highly dependent on the wood products industry which accounts for 8,600 workers. Other major industries included agriculture (tenth among Oregon's counties), transportation, trade and services and manufacturing (food products, metals, machinery, plastics and electronic instruments).

Hospitals, medical groups and physicians. As was mentioned earlier, Sacred Heart Hospital in Eugene was part of the Health and Hospital Services, a Catholic system sponsored by the Sisters of St. Joseph of Peace.

The McKinsey Williamette Hospital, a 125-bed facility, located in the neighboring community of Springfield, is a competitor of Sacred Heart. Most of the physicians in Lane County were credentialed at both hospitals.

The Eugene Clinic, with approximately 60 physicians, was the largest clinic in the area. Close to half of the clinic's physicians were in primary care. Physicians at the Eugene Clinic tended to admit most of their patients to Sacred Heart Hospital for inpatient services.

Up until the mid-1980s, the Lane County medical community could be characterized as collegial; competition was minimal. According to Robert Crist, MD, one of the founders of the Oregon Medical Group, most physicians were doing well financially and enjoying the practice of medicine. However, he said this tranquil environment was shattered by events, such as the growth in the HMO population in Lane County, the purchase of medical groups by hospitals, the threat of Kaiser Permanente coming into the area, and the formation of the Oregon Medical Group.

Lane Independent Practice Association. The Lane IPA was an important part of the development of the health care delivery system in the county from the late 1970s through early 1993. The formation of the IPA was related to community pressure to form an HMO, SelectCare. This federally-qualified HMO needed a delivery system and the IPA was formed to provide such a mechanism. Nearly all of the 450 physicians in Lane County joined the IPA and became part of the HMO provider panel.

According to Mark Litchman, MD, a family practice physician who came to Eugene in the late 1970s, "Up until 1983, the IPA's payment system worked fine. Participating physicians received the withhold at the end of the year, sometimes even more than the 15 percent. But then the withhold began to decrease and finally evaporated; we weren't doing a good job of controlling utilization." (The IPA covered between 20,000 and 25,000 lives when these problems surfaced in the early 1980s.)

In response to a continuing decline in the financial fortunes of the IPA, in 1986 several primary care physicians proposed that the IPA capitate a group of primary doctors in order to gain control of utilization. (The IPA was paid on a capitated basis but, as noted, individual physicians were paid on a discounted fee-for-service basis; there were inadequate incentives or controls to limit utilization.) This proposal led to a controversial meeting of the IPA membership and a decision not to capitate primary care physicians. According to several primary care physicians who participated in the meeting, it was very well attended ("we saw people we hadn't seen in years"), and many physicians, both primary care and specialists alike, left this meeting frustrated and angry. This decision by the IPA membership was one the factors contributing to the formation of the Oregon Medical Group (see discussion later in this case study).

In 1993 the Lane IPA was still operating and had responsibility for more than 58,000 lives. Physicians continued to be paid on a discounted fee-for-service basis with a potential 15 percent withhold; however, funds were usually not available to pay the withhold.

Growth of managed care. In Eugene the initial impetus for the formation of an HMO came from local residents, including several persons associated with the University of Oregon. With the benefit of a federal grant, SelectCare was established in 1978.

Because of over-utilization, poor economic conditions in the Eugene area and inexperienced management, SelectCare ran into financial troubles in 1982. Sacred Heart purchased the HMO in 1983; at that time it had 10,000 subscribers.

Dr. Litchman had served as medical director of the HMO for several years, including the early 1980s and since the acquisition of SelectCare by Sacred Heart.   He reported that the HMO had expanded to three additional counties and had 65,000 subscribers.   In addition to a commercial product, the HMO offered a Medicare supplemental package (around 6,000 subscribers) and a Medicaid-risk product (3,000 participants).

Capital Health Care based in Salem, which was owned by Blue Cross & Blue Shield of Oregon, had 15,000 subscribers in Lane County. Capital offered both commercial and Medicare products.

Sacred Heart Health System

Sacred Heart Health System (SHHS) was formed to coordinate the various aspects of health care delivery and financing in Lane County and surrounding areas. It included Sacred Heart Hospital, SelectCare (the HMO) and the physician component. SHHS was designed to facilitate the integration of services.

Sacred Heart Hospital.   With just under 1,900 employees, the hospital was the largest private employer in Lane County. The hospital had 450 staffed beds and operated at 65.5 percent of capacity in 1992.

Exhibit B shows several indicators of volume, including inpatient admissions and patient days for the hospital, for the period of 1988 through 1992. As these data indicate, the hospital has performed well in the face of the general decline in inpatient activities.

EXHIBIT B.
Indicators of Volume, Sacred Heart
Health System, 1988-1992

Indicator	1988	1989	1990	1991	1992
Total Revenue (millions)	$95.3	$116.4	$128.1	$146.3	$157.9
Expenses (millions)	85.2	104.3	119.8	138.4	150.1
Net Earnings (millions)	$11.5	$11.7	$9.8	$8.0	$10.7
Patient Encounters* (thousands)	25.2	27.6	28.8	28.9	28.9
Number of Employees	1,694	1,779	1,919	1,981	1,860

Source: Sacred Heart Health System, July, 1993.
* Inpatient adjusted admissions. Outpatient visits increased from 90,000 in 1988 to 143,877 in 1992.

The hospital was in sound financial condition with assets of $206.8 million, liabilities of $23.7 million and a net worth of $183.1 million as of the end of 1992.

SelectCare. A brief history of SelectCare, including its purchase by Sacred Heart, was outlined earlier. In 1993, SelectCare represented approximately 15,000 patients of the Oregon Medical Group.

Physicians. Under the leadership of Wesley Jacobs, MD, Vice President of Medical Affairs, the system has started a number of different initiatives involving physicians, including the Oregon Medical Group, the Lane IPA and relationships with specific physicians and groups that participate on the hospital medical staff. The role of the Physician Practice Board is discussed later in this case study.

The Formation of the Oregon Medical Group (OMG)

Events leading to the formation of OMG.   Dr. Crist told us, "A bunch of us were sitting around having a beer after a tennis match and we were speculating about the health care system of the future.   We talked about where medicine was headed and the growing disparity between primary care and specialists' earnings. We were frustrated over our inability to recruit new primary care physicians. We recognized that Eugene had been an island in a managed care environment, and we thought this would change. In addition, we were very concerned that Kaiser might come in. In fact, at one time they announced they were coming to Eugene."

Dr. Jacobs, who at one time practiced as a cardiologist, was present at this initial informal session. He explained, "We started out by talking about how to achieve world peace but then began talking about health care. We were aware that few, if any, new primary care physicians were coming into the community. We did not see replacements for the fine primary care physicians we already had. We were concerned about how much longer fee-for-service medicine would survive. It smelled like change was in the wind."

He went on, "From a hospital perspective, we knew that to be well positioned for the future we needed a strong primary care base. Therefore, we needed to have a way to attract and retain primary care doctors. The job was not getting done back in the mid-1980s."

When the various primary care groups decided to proceed with the formation of OMG, the major motivating factors were positioning for managed care contracting, improving physician income and attracting and retaining primary care physicians. According to Dr. Crist, "The initial planning called for the inclusion of specialists, primarily to help share the overhead and help make the practice economically viable."

Jim Schwering, Executive Director of the Oregon Medical Services Organization (OMSO), was not present at these initial meetings. However, in reviewing the situation in the mid-1980s he said that two things were happening:

(1)   There was a clear decline in economics for primary care physicians. Hospital executives also realized that if nothing was done about the potential primary care physician crisis, the

hospital would be at the whim of third party payers. If there was an insufficient primary care physician supply, the patient base of the hospital would probably also diminish.

(2) Delivery systems were changing in Oregon, with managed care becoming an increasing percentage of every physician's practice mix. Oregon is a state with a significant number of managed care products. An increasing amount of the welfare system is served by capitated managed care plans.

The role of the hospital. From the beginning, Sacred Heart Hospital supported the effort to form a medical group. One physician in the Oregon Medical Group said that following the IPA's rejection of the proposal to capitate a group of primary care doctors, "We went to Sister Monica (the CEO of Health and Hospital Services) and worked out an action plan. Dr. Jacobs was part of these discussions. We discussed what the hospital and primary care docs might do together."

In terms of selling the Sacred Heart Hospital board on investing in the development of a medical group, Dr. Jacobs said, "We convinced them of the same factors we discussed earlier — an eroding primary care base in the community spelled trouble for the hospital, and that solo practitioners would not be able to make it as the health care system moved more into a capitated environment. They could see the need for something like this and agreed that the hospital should support it financially to the extent possible."

Wayne Atwood, a wood products executive and member of the board of both Sacred Heart Health System and the Oregon MSO, said, "When Oregon Medical Group was formed, all hell broke loose among the medical staff. Some of the specialists accused the hospital of showing preferential treatment to a small group of primary care physicians."

Nevertheless, the board of the hospital decided to pursue the idea, and agreed to fund studies of the concept. A consulting firm was retained to examine the various organizational models for the group practice and the hospital.

Selecting a model. According to Dr. Crist, the consultants were instrumental in getting physicians and the hospital to agree that a management services organization (MSO) model was best. "Our physicians were unwilling, and in many cases unable, to contribute their personal capital. We also wanted to maintain our independence from the hospital. The MSO model allowed us to gain access to capital through the sale of certain assets, such as equipment (several groups retained ownership of their buildings, and the individual physicians and groups kept their accounts receivable). It was also apparent that whatever we did we could not continue to require a heavy buy-in if we hoped to attract new primary care physicians."

Schwering said, "The group looked at other alternatives to the MSO but there really weren't many options available at the time the Oregon Medical Group and the Oregon MSO were formed. Essentially, there were three options: employ physicians, create a foundation or create an MSO. At the time the management services organization was the preferred organizational structure."

Working out the initial financing. The initial investment in establishing the Oregon MSO was around $5 million. This money was used for working capital, the purchase of equipment, building two new practice sites and equipping new offices adjacent to the hospital. It also helped with the expenses of organizing the new group (e.g., consolidated accounting and billing systems, standardizing forms).

Dr. Jacobs said that the consultant who assisted in putting the group together emphasized the need for supplemental income to support primary care physicians in the group. "He made it clear that the savings from consolidating practices and centralizing administrative functions wouldn't be enough to make this new venture worthwhile. We talked about the need for ancillary services and income, especially laboratory and X-ray. Of course, we hoped that being able to access managed care contracts would bring in more income."

Launching the new organization. Two years after making a preliminary decision to proceed, including the signing of letters of intent, the OMG was formed effective November 1, 1988. In reflecting on the time it took to get OMG organized, Dr. Crist said, "We probably could have done it faster. There wasn't the pressure that many organizations are facing today."

Even while the OMG and MSO were organizing, one of the original medical groups that had participated in all of the meetings and done everything but sign a letter of intent, decided to sell to McKinsey Williamette Hospital. According to one physician in OMG, "It is pretty well known around the community that the hospital paid these doctors $250,000 each to join with them."

The individual medical groups were dissolved, and each participating physician paid $1,000 for one share and one vote in the new for-profit Oregon Medical Group. Most physicians continued to practice at the same locations in which they had practiced before formation of OMG.

Issues of integrating the different medical practices. Jim Schwering noted that the problems of integrating the practices were complex and required extreme patience to work out. "We had different patient sign-in forms, different billing forms, different policies on collections and different pay scales for our staff. We had different pension plans, and this posed some of the most difficult problems. Some of the physicians wanted to retain the assets in their plans, and others did not."

He went on, "We really had to teach physicians how to work together as part of an organization. We all had to become accustomed to having a governing board and operating like a business."

Dr. Litchman added, "We were seven different groups and we did everything differently. Melding us together was a major hurdle but one that was not insurmountable. We had to change our thinking; we had to adapt a broader perspective. We have come a long way, but some of us still think of ourselves as part of one of the original medical groups rather than being in Oregon Medical Group."

Adding specialists. According to Virginia Slate, Assistant Administrator, Sacred Heart Hospital and Chairperson, OMSO, the matter of specialists was, and is, a controversial issue. "When OMG was conceived, there was talk of bringing in specialists, primarily to help cover the costs of primary care. The hospital board was confused on whether specialists were to be in the group or not. The issue of adding specialists to OMG came up again two years ago, and the independent specialists at Sacred Heart went nuts. I can't tell you how upset they were and, of course, it went right to the board. We had to ask OMG to hold off on this move."

Dr. Crist said, "We had some surgeons ready to come into OMG. They were ready to sign on the dotted line, but we agreed to delay this action. These surgeons have since joined in forming another medical group."

The SHHS administration asked OMG to hold off on this matter until the strategic planning process could be completed. This effort, called Mission 2000, is discussed later. At the time of the preparation of this case study, no decision had been made relative to adding specialists to OMG.

Laboratory and radiology. Both OMSO and OMG had originally hoped to generate ancillary income through ownership of and use of a laboratory and of radiology equipment (primarily X-ray). However, specific proposals to the OMSO board conflicted with Sacred Heart's prior agreements with pathologists and radiologists, and it was necessary for OMSO to pull back. Slate said, "In a sense, the hospital took away these physicians' right to generate supplemental income through ancillaries. By joining with us they cut themselves off from an income source that is critically important to most successful primary care groups. This was part of their original business plan and it was a blow to the group when they found they couldn't proceed."

She continued, "I felt, and others in hospital management agreed, that we had to find ways to assist these physicians financially. We are now covering some of the expenses associated with recruiting." She added that it is very difficult for a non-profit hospital to assist physicians without running afoul of private inurement laws. "I've lost several nights' sleep over these kinds of issues. These are sensitive matters."

Summary of activity, 1989 through 1993. Exhibit C is a summary of key indicators for the OMG. The data on this exhibit show that total revenues more than doubled between 1989 and 1993, and that the number of patient visits increased from 111,000 to 196,500 over the five-year period (see Exhibit D).

In terms of cost effectiveness, the average charge per patient has increased from $66 to $80 over the five years, up four percent per year.

The productivity of physicians associated with OMG has increased over the five years, growing from 3,800 patient visits in 1989 to 4,300 in 1993, up 13 percent. Net income for physicians had increased from $92,000 per full-time equivalent in 1989 to $128,800 in 1993, a 40 percent gain in five years.

Governance

Oregon Medical Group. OMG was governed by a seven-person board of directors. Board members were elected by the shareholders for three-year terms which were staggered. The board met monthly.

EXHIBIT C.
Key Indicators, Oregon Medical Group, P.C.
Eugene, Oregon 1989-1993

Indicator	1989	1990	1991	1992	Projected 1993
Total Charges (Production)	$7,315,225	$9,439,816	$12,988,462	$14,160,694	$15,722,640
Total Operating Net Revenue	$6,396,055	$8,960,468	$11,413,657	$12,059,832	$13,832,160
Operating Expenses	3,709,712	5,376,281	6,791,126	7,175,600	7,970,435
Net Income From Operations	2,686,343	3,584,187	4,622,531	4,884,232	5,861,725
FTE Physicians	29.25	31.25	38.75	40.75	45.40
Average Charges Per FTE	$250,093	$302,074	$335,186	$347,502	$345,553
Average Revenue Per FTE	218,669	286,735	294,546	295,947	304,004
Net Income per FTE	91,841	114,694	119,291	119,858	128,829
Patient Visits per FTE	3,800	4,074	4,249	4,295	4,319
Patient Visits	111,150	127,314	164,637	175,029	196,533
Average Charge Per Patient	$65.81	$74.15	$78.89	$80.90	$80.00
Average Revenue Per Patient	57.54	70.38	69.33	68.90	70.38

Source: Oregon Medical Group, P.C., June, 1993.

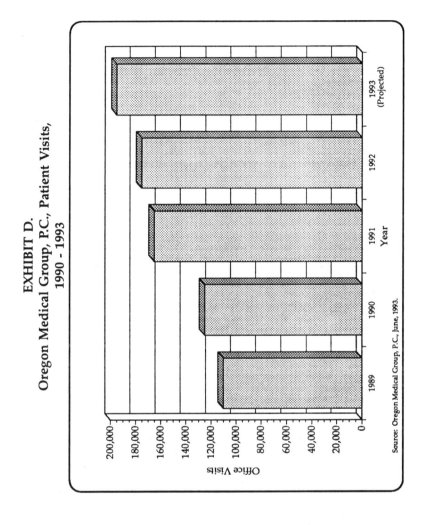

EXHIBIT D.
Oregon Medical Group, P.C., Patient Visits,
1990 - 1993

Source: Oregon Medical Group, P.C., June, 1993.

According to Jim Schwering, "One of the things that OMG did right was giving each physician shareholder one vote. There is a one-year waiting period for new doctors before they are eligible to become shareholders, so you can see they are forced into decision making very quickly. I think this is much better than having a small group of physicians own the organization with a large of number of physician employees."

Oregon MSO. This organization was governed by an eight-member board, four from the hospital (two non-physician hospital board members and two hospital administrators) and four physicians from the OMG. Members of the OMSO board were also elected for three-year terms (staggered so that there are new board members elected every year). It requires three "yes" votes from both hospital and physician members to make a decision.

Virginia Slate said, "The chairman for the first three years was Dr. Crist. We had an agreement that the chairperson would serve a three-year term, and that the position would alternate between representatives of OMG and Sacred Heart."

Slate, who was educated as a registered nurse and was involved in the mid-1980s in managing the Eugene Clinic, said that she spends five or six hours each week in business relating to the OMSO. "But, there have been times when it required half my time."

Schwering said that Slate is ideally qualified to head up the OMSO board. "She is a nurse and the physicians have a special respect for her because of her clinical background. And, because of her experience with the Eugene Clinic, she understands medical group practices and how running them differs from hospital administration. She is a valuable asset to our organization."

Physician-Hospital Integration in Eugene

Mission 2000. In January, 1990, the SHHS board held a retreat focusing on the future of health care. Dr. Jacobs said, "As a result of that meeting we developed a template, or rough skeleton, of what we could see coming and what we need to do to respond. We concluded that there needed to be substantial integration of our physicians, our HMO (SelectCare) and Sacred Heart Hospital."

Following the retreat, the System engaged in a nine-month strategic planning process leading up to the preparation of a plan called "Mission 2000." Dr. Jacobs noted that development of the plan involved an in-depth analysis of the situation, including emphasis on the factors driving costs for the System. Part of this analysis included field visits to a number of large clinics and integrated delivery systems around the country (e.g., Mayo Clinic, Virginia Mason). "We wanted to know how much cost we could take out of the system. We concluded that if we could do everything right, we might be able to reduce costs by 20 to 25 percent."

Dr. Jacobs continued, "I'm not talking only about the hospital. These savings could only be generated by gaining control of the whole health care delivery and financing system. For example, some of these savings would come from cutting administrative expenses associated with health insurance. Obviously, we needed to align our financial incentives throughout the system."

Every strategic initiative considered as part of the planning process had to satisfy three criteria: reduces costs, improves access and enhances quality of care. "If a strategy only satisfied two of these criteria, we dropped it; it had to satisfy all three. When we went through this process the increasingly important role of primary care physicians stood out since they are vital in controlling costs, providing access and enhancing quality."

Dr. Jacobs said that many of the specialists were apprehensive about this plan, and a few were very upset. "Once again, we stirred up a hornets' nest. However, with the 1992 Presidential election, and the advent of health care reform, things have cooled down."

Physician Practice Board. As a result of the plan, the Physician Practice Board was formed in early 1992. Within Sacred Heart Health System, it functioned at the same level as SelectCare and Sacred Heart Hospital. Exhibit E is an organizational chart showing how the Physician Practice Board fits into the SHHS structure.

The Board was made up of seven physicians who were appointed by the System board; Dr. Jacobs was chairman. He said, "This is totally different from the medical staff. This is the business arm of the hospital and physicians who use Sacred Heart. We can recommend actions to the System board. We maintain a panel of physicians and set the policies on the distribution of funds from the various risk pools. As you can see

EXHIBIT E.
Sacred Heart Health System (SHHS)

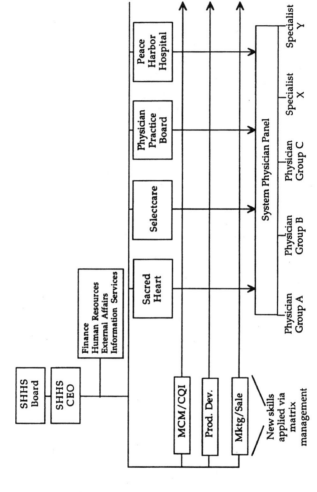

Source: Sacred Heart Health System, June, 1993.

from the organization chart, we are also involved in continuous quality improvement (CQI), product development, marketing and sales."

In terms of selecting physicians to be part of the panel, Dr. Jacobs said that nearly all specialists were included. "To participate, primary care physicians have to meet several criteria: They must be in a group, have an information system, be willing to accept risk and have the ability to perform utilization review and quality assurance. Only Oregon Medical Group and the Eugene Clinic have been able to meet these criteria."

On this latter point, Schwering said that the inclusion of OMG as one of two primary care groups in the panel was the result of OMG's ability to prove its cost effectiveness in the delivery of care. "Three years ago studies showed that health care in Eugene was five to 10 percent more expensive than Portland. However, I was recently told by a representative of a large HMO that we — the Oregon Medical Group — were five percent below Portland."

Information Systems

Dr. Jacobs said that the need to revamp the system's information system is imperative to being able to integrate physicians and perform well in a managed care environment. "We will be spending around $25 million on this over the next three years." Dr. Jacobs went on, "Hospital boards are going to have to quit spending so much on bricks and mortar and technology and spend more on information systems and the support of primary care physicians."

Major Accomplishments

Schwering noted several accomplishments of the OMG and OMSO. "First, we dramatically improved our facilities, including construction of two new offices. We consolidated several groups and individual physicians into what is now a 17-person internal medicine group in the medical office building adjacent to Sacred Heart. We also have a women's clinic on the first floor of the building."

He also said the group has made great progress in learning to work together as an organization; that a corporate culture of cooperation was developing. "Many of our systems have been streamlined and we handle a huge volume of patients and paperwork with a relatively small staff.

The long-term viability of this group is not dependent on a single person; we have systems in place and people trained to carry on."

He also noted the growth of the group — from 24 physicians in 1988 to 57 in early 1993. Other indicators of the growth of the medical group were included in Exhibit C.

Virginia Slate agreed that the improvement in medical offices was one of the major accomplishments. "In addition, we have professional management, a quality assurance system, and a much more streamlined operation. Some of the physicians' office equipment and procedures were badly in need of upgrading. One practice had a 20-year old telephone system, and we are talking about the need for sophisticated on-line access to clinical and patient information!"

Dr. Jacobs said that both Oregon Medical Group and Sacred Heart Health System were well positioned for growth in managed care and for health care reform. "We are way ahead of where we would be if we hadn't made this decision in 1988 to move ahead with the formation of OMG."

Dr. Jacobs also said that the presence of OMG definitely helped attain the goal of attracting and retaining more primary care physicians. "As I mentioned earlier, the lack of new primary care physicians coming into the community in the mid-1980s concerned us a lot. OMG has helped turn this situation around." Dr. Crist added, "OMG has facilitated recruiting. Most new physicians want good management and guaranteed salaries. They don't want the hassles of setting up their own practices."

Several individuals interviewed said that OMG was a low-cost provider. Dr. Crist said, "Even though only 25 to 30 percent of our business is capitated, we made a decision that we were going to run our practice like the entire business was at risk. This was the right decision for the long term but it has certainly taken its toll on our incomes in the short run."

On this same point, Slate noted that OMG was part of a risk pool for SelectCare, and that the organization's performance was substantially better than that of other physicians. "This provides evidence that as we get more heavily into capitation, OMG will be very cost competitive."

Wayne Atwood, who was on the board of the OMSO, summarized the accomplishments this way: "Formation of OMG helped our primary care physicians compete for managed care contracts, their practices have become more efficient and modern and the new group is definitely a low-cost provider, well positioned for the future."

Lessons Learned

Dr. Crist explained that one of the most important lessons learned was to hire a group practice administrator at the beginning. "We waited too long before we brought in Jim Schwering. We could have saved ourselves a lot of grief if we had brought him in earlier. For one thing we made a major error in the type of computer system we installed. Somehow or other in the hassle of putting the groups together, and the continuing uncertainty over whether we were really going to be able to pull it off, we neglected the important step of identifying and hiring a manager."

Dr. Litchman said that you don't win any popularity contests with fellow physicians when you do something like forming a large group practice. "The formation of OMG created anxiety and fear. Until we came along, Kaiser Permanente was the bogey man; everyone was afraid they would come in. But, when we got started, this focused the attention on us. You need to recognize that you will feel the ill will of your colleagues if you try something like this."

Wayne Atwood believes that realizing economies of scale by combining a number of small practices is questionable. "You wouldn't do this just to save dollars."

Virginia Slate commented that the lessons learned from her perspective as a hospital administrator were:

(1) "The medical group must have a representative on the governing board of the hospital. This is needed to facilitate communication and an understanding of the new physician group.

(2) Explain the animal — the Oregon MSO — over and over again to hospital managers and the board. This is the biggest mistake we made. Make it so clear that the board could pass a quiz on it.

(3) More cross pollination between senior level executives of the hospital and medical group. We should have brought Jim Schwering into the fabric of the organization. One example of the differences in understanding involves physician recruiting. Our hospital board members think that recruiting doctors means paying moving expenses. They don't realize the extent of the financial commitment necessary to bring new primary care physicians into the community.

(4) Before a deal is made, it is important to find out more about the way physicians operate in their offices, the nature of their existing equipment and systems and any special problems that we might anticipate. There were some surprises out there."

Issues for the Future

One of the challenges of the future for Oregon Medical Group is to develop a system of referrals to specialists. In early 1993 this issue had not yet been tackled. But, as Dr. Litchman said, "The continuing growth of capitated contracts, and our willingness to take on risk, is going to force us into being selective in our use of specialists. Some long-time friendships and referral patterns are likely to be broken, and this will be painful."

Low compensation for some OMG physicians was an important issue in early 1993. According to Dr. Crist, the average income for primary care physicians (excluding three obstetricians who earned more) was $80,000 in 1992. When you have to pay more than this to recruit new family practice docs, it is inequitable. We are going to have to figure out some ways to improve compensation."

Virginia Slate said, "Despite the problems, I think we have made tremendous progress. You know this group is now the 800-pound gorilla of the health care system here in Lane County. We know that the future of health care is highly dependent on primary care, and we have a large group of primary care physicians organized, working together and poised for the future. It was a visionary thing to do."

---

* Jim Schwering, Executive Director, and his staff made this case study possible by arranging for interviews and providing background data. We appreciated their help.

Case Study #8
GEISINGER
Danville, Pennsylvania

— Persons Interviewed —

Stuart Heydt, MD, President, Geisinger Foundation
F. K. Ackerman, Jr., Senior Vice President, Operations/Central Region
Laurence H. Beck, MD, Executive Vice President, Clinical Program
    and Process Improvement
Ernest Campbell, MD, Family Practice, Bloomsburg GMG
Keith T. Coleman, Senior Vice President, Finance/Geisinger System
    Chief Financial Officer
Robert Haddad, MD, Senior Vice President and Medical Director,
    Community Practice, Central Region
Jack M. Hartman, Esquire, Senior Vice President, Legal Services
Howard Hughes, MD, Senior Vice President, Geisinger Health Plan
Charles Laubach, MD, Director Emeritus, Cardiology
O. Fred Miller, MD, Director, Dermatology
William C. Reed, Senior Vice President, Operations/Geisinger System
    Chief Information Officer
Robert C. Spahr, MD, Senior Vice President, Clinical Operations
    Central Region
Theodore E. Townsend, Senior Vice President, Marketing Operations
Frank J. Trembulak, Executive Vice President, Operations
David K. Wessner, Executive Vice President, Program and
    Process Improvement
Gary L. Wolfgang, MD, Chairman, Division of Surgery

July, 1993

EXHIBIT A.
Location of Danville, Wilkes Barre and Harrisburg in Pennsylvania and Geisinger System Regions

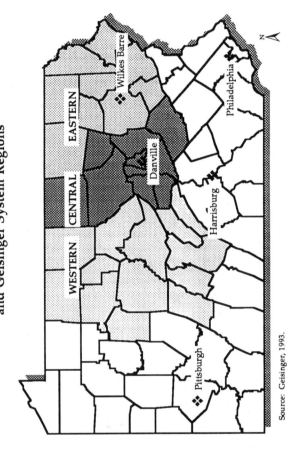

Source: Geisinger, 1993.

GEISINGER*
Danville, Pennsylvania

The Geisinger health care system included a large multispecialty clinic (more than 500 physicians), two acute care hospitals (577-bed Geisinger Medical Center in Danville and 230-bed Wyoming Valley Medical Center near Wilkes-Barre), more than 40 network sites, mainly staffed by primary care physicians, the largest HMO in rural America with 145,000 members, a medical education and research foundation, a substance abuse facility, a nursing training program and other health care services.

The Geisinger health care system had more than 7,600 employees and accounted for nearly 1.2 million patient visits in 1992. Net revenues that year exceeded $460 million.

The Geisinger Health Care Marketplace

Geisinger served a population of 2.3 million persons living within a 20,000-square mile area of central and northeastern Pennsylvania. The Geisinger system's service area included 31 of Pennsylvania's 67 counties. Exhibit A is a map of Pennsylvania showing the location of Danville, Wilkes-Barre (the site of the second acute care hospital and a large Geisinger medical group), Harrisburg, Philadelphia and Pittsburgh. Exhibit A also shows Geisinger's three regions.

The hospital, clinic and related facilities are on a 430-acre site in Danville, a community of 7,000 residents. Danville is located in the Appalachian Range, near the Susquehanna River. Interstate Highway #80 is adjacent to the community and is an important factor extending the service area to the east and west. As noted, Geisinger has outpatient facilities at more than 40 sites and a hospital in Wilkes-Barre, 60 miles northeast of Danville.

Demographics of service area. Residents of the Geisinger service area were older than the state and national averages, with a much higher proportion on Medicare. Income levels were below the Pennsylvania and US averages; Medicaid covered a higher than normal proportion of residents in the service area.

Competition. There was a large number of hospitals, independent physicians and small medical groups within the 31-county Geisinger service area. In addition, major hospitals and health care systems located in Hershey (1.5 hours south), Philadelphia (three hours southeast) and Harrisburg (1.5 hours south) competed with Geisinger.

The impact of increased competition on the fringes of Geisinger's service area was reflected in the 1990 to 1992 drop in the proportion of admissions to the system from outlying counties (see later discussion).

Frank Trembulak, Executive Vice President for Operations, told us that the attitudes of physicians and hospitals in the service area toward Geisinger had changed in the past year or so. "They are more interested in collaboration today, and we are always willing to talk with them. Our ability to work together depends on their motivations, and whether or not we can agree on what it is going to take to succeed in the future." He noted that if a physician group or hospital was primarily interested in preserving its present situation, collaboration probably wouldn't work. "However, if they are genuinely interested in finding ways to meet the needs of people in their area, we probably have a basis for further discussion."

Health plan coverage patterns/payor mix. Because of the demographics of people living in the service area, the payment sources for a large portion of the patients were relatively poor. Medicare represented nearly 37 percent of the gross revenues of Geisinger and a higher percentage of the patients served. Medicaid accounted for nearly 10 percent of Geisinger's gross revenues in 1992.

The Geisinger Health Plan, an HMO serving approximately seven percent of the residents of the area in 1993, accounted for 19 percent of Geisinger's gross revenues. Blue Cross (two different regional systems) was the major private insurer, accounting for 11 percent; Blue Shield represented five percent of Geisinger's gross revenues. Other commercial insurance and self-pay constituted 18 percent of the system's gross revenues.

Patient origin/market share. It was estimated that in 1993 Geisinger captured around five percent of the total health care business — physician visits, outpatient procedures and inpatient admissions — originating in the service area. However, market share in nearby counties was in the 50 to 80 percent range.

The proportion of patients originating in the smaller 18-county primary service area represented 92.5 percent of Geisinger's patients in 1992 (year ending June 30). The proportion coming from these areas had increased from 86.3 percent two years earlier. In other words, although Geisinger served individuals within 31 counties, the proportion of its patients coming from the smaller primary service area was increasing.

Geisinger primary care physicians represented just under 10 percent of all primary care physicians practicing in the 31-county service area.

History of Geisinger

In 1912, Abigail A. Geisinger, then 85 years old, met with three of her fellow townspeople in the parlor of her home in Danville and advised them that she would furnish $500,000 to build a "modern" hospital. She gave the men this charge: "Make my hospital right; make it the best."

The 63-bed hospital opened in 1915 during a typhoid fever epidemic and recorded 761 admissions during its first 12 months. The hospital was named after Abigail Geisinger's late husband, George F. Geisinger, who had earned his fortune in coal mining. (In 1961 the name of the hospital was changed to the "Geisinger Medical Center.")

In what proved to be a key decision, Abigail Geisinger retained Harold Foss, MD, a young surgeon trained at the Mayo Clinic, as the hospital's first physician. Dr. Foss persuaded her that the hospital should be organized as a full-time group practice following the Mayo Clinic model. Dr. Foss proceeded to recruit physicians who were disposed to work as part of a multispecialty group on a salaried basis. F. Kenneth Ackerman, Jr., Senior Vice President, Operations/Central Region, said this decision made a huge difference in the organization's future. "I am convinced that if Mrs. Geisinger had decided that the hospital and medical staff should develop along traditional lines, we would be looking today at a 50-bed facility with 20 physicians on the medical staff."

The initial governing board of the hospital and clinic consisted of businessmen and clergymen from Danville. However, dissatisfaction with the "limited vision" of the board prompted Abigail Geisinger and Dr. Foss to approach the Scranton Trust Company (later a part of Northeastern Bank of Pennsylvania which was acquired by PNC, a large banking company, in 1993). The bank managers convinced Abigail Geisinger that she should execute an irrevocable deed of trust, transferring the hospital and all of its assets to the bank to be administered according to the stipulations in her deed.

Mrs. Geisinger died in 1921 at the age of 94, leaving an additional endowment to the hospital.

Leadership and management. The founding physician, Dr. Foss, was the head of Geisinger for 43 years. He was followed by Leonard Bush, MD, an orthopedic surgeon, who was president from 1958 to 1974, a span of 16 years. Henry Hood, MD, a neurosurgeon, became president in 1974 and held that office until 1990 (16 years) when he retired. The fourth president, Stuart Heydt, MD, took office in 1990.

Geisinger's management style was to pair a physician with an administrator to manage important elements of the Geisinger system. For example, Robert Spahr, MD and Kenneth Ackerman jointly managed the Central Region; this included management of the Geisinger Medical Center, the 350 physicians in the region and other activities. Laurence Beck, MD, and David Wessner jointly managed the clinical and process improvement programs. Frank Trembulak said that the concept of a physician and administrator teaming to manage a group was championed by Dr. Hood. "Dr. Hood recognized that Geisinger had to operate more like a business."

The Department of Health decision. One of the major regulatory decisions affecting Geisinger occurred in 1978 when the hospital received authorization to proceed with a major expansion program. At the same time, the State Department of Health designated Geisinger Medical Center as one of four tertiary care hospitals in the Commonwealth of Pennsylvania.

During the same period, Geisinger physicians and administrators had been working with a group in Wilkes-Barre who wanted to establish a clinic and hospital in that metropolitan area. However, according to Kenneth Ackerman, "The group could not get its financing together and they asked us to take over the project. We did, and that led to the construction of the 230-bed hospital and the establishment of a multispecialty group adjacent to the hospital." (The Wilkes-Barre hospital had an open staff; approximately one third of the admissions originated from independent physicians.)

Building programs. The Geisinger facilities in Danville have undergone numerous expansion programs, increasing the capacity to 577 inpatient beds, with space for an outpatient clinic staffed by 300 physicians (the remaining 200 physicians were in Wilkes-Barre and at the other locations within the service area). In 1993, the Danville facility was being expanded once again with the addition of the 86-bed Janet Weis Children's Hospital. In 1993, the Geisinger Medical Center had 17 operating rooms, an emergency department that treated more than 35,000 patients annually and departments for oncology, open-heart surgery and nearly all medical specialties.

Geisinger's Recent Growth and Driving Strategies

Geisinger's mission and driving strategies. Geisinger's mission was, "To improve the health of the people of the Commonwealth through an integrated system of health services based on a balanced program of patient care, education, and research."

To accomplish its mission, Geisinger adopted four "driving strategies" which were referred to frequently by physician leaders and others during the interview process as part of the preparation of this case study. The four strategies, which evolved beginning in 1991, are:

- Function as a single organization.

- Clinical programs and clinical process improvements size and drive the system.

- Managed care is our primary business strategy.

- Seek collaborative opportunities to increase access to services in a cost-effective manner.

Geisinger did not have a formal strategic plan prior to 1992. Frank Trembulak said that whenever he talked to Dr. Hood about Geisinger's strategic plan, "He would say that we had one. Then he would pull out a single sheet of paper with three or four bullets on it. In his mind, planning restricted our options, and he wanted Geisinger to be flexible, to be able to take advantage of opportunities."

The Geisinger physician group. In 1993, the Geisinger Clinic existed in the corporate structure, but did not function as a separate entity. For example, the 350 physicians in the Central Division were part of a group that included the Geisinger Medical Center; there was no separate physician organization.

The number of Geisinger physicians increased from 207 in 1982 to 499 in 1992. The increase has been steady over the 10-year period (see Exhibit B).

Physician staff at the main campus in Danville increased from 174 in 1982 to 283 in 1992, a 63 percent increase. Medical staff at other locations increased from 33 to 216 during the same period, up 555 percent in 10 years. The proportion of primary care physicians had increased steadily over the past decade to the point where these types of doctors represented 25 to 30 percent of the total.

The number of patient visits to Geisinger physicians increased from more than 991,000 in 1988 to more than 1,198,000 in 1992.

Geisinger's acute care hospitals. Exhibit C shows several indicators of volume for the Geisinger Medical Center for the 1988 through 1992 period.

Exhibit C.
Admissions, Average Length of Stay, Inpatient Days and Other Indicators, Geisinger Medical Center, Fiscal Year 1988 to 1992

	1988	1989	1990	1991	1992
Discharges	20,036	20,001	20,082	19,668	20,089
Patient Days	152,539	154,829	156,641	158,532	159,647
Length of Stay	7.5	7.8	7.8	8.1	8.0
Occupancy	73.2%	73.5%	74.4%	75.3%	75.6%
Inpatient Surgical Procedures	9,059	9,236	8,726	8,620	8,914
Outpatient Surgeries	4,982	5,466	6,340	6,810	7,538
Medicare Case Mix Index	1.4882	1.5360	1.6050	1.6240	1.7038

Note: Discharges, patient days, length of stay and occupancy figures exclude nursery.

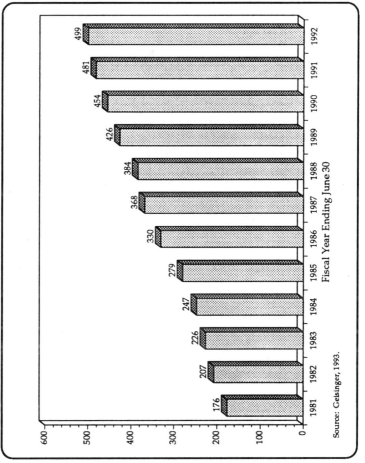

EXHIBIT B.
Number of Geisinger Clinic Physicians

Source: Geisinger, 1993.

The Geisinger Wyoming Valley Medical Center in Wilkes-Barre has shown a slight downward trend in discharges and patient days over the 1988-to-1992 period. However, occupancy rates were 70 percent or higher during the previous five years.

Through its health plan, Geisinger has relationships with 23 additional community hospitals in the service area. These hospitals care for about 10 percent of the inpatient admissions generated by GHP subscribers.

Geisinger did not push its physicians in remote locations to refer their patients to the Geisinger Medical Center; doctors were free to use local hospitals. In fact, one Geisinger physician was chief of staff of the hospital in Bloomsburg, eight miles from Danville. Frank Trembulak said, "We believe that routine hospital services should be provided as close to home as possible. Also, Geisinger Medical Center is a tertiary care facility, and its costs are naturally higher than those in the smaller hospitals."

Financial performance of the Geisinger system. In its 1992 fiscal year, Geisinger earned $23 million on operations and another $10 million in non-operating income (total of $33 million). That was on revenues of $413 million (charges were $650 million, indicating the large proportion of discounts and allowances in 1992). Exhibit D shows the trend in revenues and profits for the 1988-through-1992 period.

**EXHIBIT D. Geisinger System Net Revenue,
Expenses and Net Income,
1988 to 1992 (fiscal year ending June 30)**

	1988	1989	1990	1991	1992
Net Revenue	$315.0	$343.4	$383.9	$415.3	$466.0
Expenses	288.2	325.0	350.7	386.9	432.9
Net Income	$26.8	$18.4	$33.2	$28.4	$33.1

Source: Geisinger 1992 <u>Annual Report,</u> page 11.

However, Geisinger experienced a financial downturn in early 1993, leading to a downsizing of the work force. According to Keith Coleman, Senior Vice President for Finance, 400 positions were eliminated. However, since many of these positions were vacant, only 160 employees lost their jobs. It was estimated that this would save the organization $9 million annually.

Major factors accounting for the lower financial performance were discounted payment by Medicare and other payors, including changes in physician payment rates. In addition, while the growth in volume was slowing, the rate of expense growth continued to increase.

Primary Care Strategies

Kenneth Ackerman recalled that when he came to Geisinger in 1964, the organization did not have family medicine and had no remote sites; all Geisinger activities were concentrated on the Danville campus. "Sometime in the late 1960s we attempted to establish family medicine, but it didn't work. We ended up disbanding the group. Then, in the early 1970s we tried again, using a physician from a smaller community in our service area. He agreed to accept the challenge provided we would establish a residency program for family medicine. That proved to be a wise suggestion because it gave family medicine the credibility and acceptance it needed."

Charles Laubach, MD, a cardiologist who has been with Geisinger many years, said that in the 1950s Geisinger became highly specialized. "The Department of Internal Medicine ceased to exist. However, this began to change in the mid-1960s, and we began to bring in family medicine in the late 1970s and early 1980s. In my opinion, the need for family medicine was linked to the Geisinger Health Plan and its need for a network of physicians."

In 1993, 25 to 30 percent of Geisinger's physicians were in primary care. Several executives of Geisinger said that the ratio was out of balance; more primary care physicians were needed. Geisinger was attempting to recruit 32 primary care doctors. A high priority in the planning and analysis being carried out by top management was to better define the physician needs of the region, and to appropriately shape the Geisinger system to meet those needs.

As noted earlier, the impetus for developing the primary care network came from the Pennsylvania Department of Health in 1978, as part of its decision to grant Geisinger Medical Center special status as a tertiary care facility.

Kenneth Ackerman said, "We had been thinking about the need to expand geographically for some time. We didn't like having all of our eggs in one basket (Danville). And, we have always drawn heavily from

Scranton and Wilkes-Barre, indicating a need to provide more convenient services in those areas."

According to Keith Coleman, the seed money for the primary care network development came from "the Danville campus." He was referring to the medical center and specialists. Coleman said that when Geisinger purchased existing practices, it paid for fixed assets, but had not paid goodwill since 1987.

Ernest Campbell, MD, a family practice physician in the Bloomsburg Geisinger Medical Group, said that many primary care physicians were interested in coming into the Geisinger system. "They are feeling threatened by managed care, they want income security, and they recognize that Geisinger practices high-quality medicine. All of these factors make Geisinger an increasingly attractive alternative even though these doctors would lose some of their independence."

Exhibit E shows the number of Geisinger physician practice sites in 1981 through 1992. The largest growth periods were in the 1985-through-1988 period, corresponding to the decision to expand the role of the Geisinger Health Plan.

Governance and Organizational Structure

From 1915, at the inception of the hospital, the George F. Geisinger Hospital was the only organization. All physicians were employees of the hospital and later Geisinger Medical Center.

1981 organizational structure. According to Kenneth Ackerman, the 1981 reorganization was significant on several counts. It created, for the first time, a separate organization for physicians -- the not-for-profit Geisinger Clinic. Ackerman said, "The regulations impacting the hospital were encroaching on our physicians. We wanted to give them more independence in terms of how they practiced and ran the business side of the clinic."

Exhibit F is the organizational chart for Geisinger for the period 1981 through December 1992. Seven of the 10 organizations were not-for-profits, and three were organized as for-profit entities.

1992 reorganization. Beginning in 1991, the leaders of Geisinger concluded that the organizational structure was leading to too much

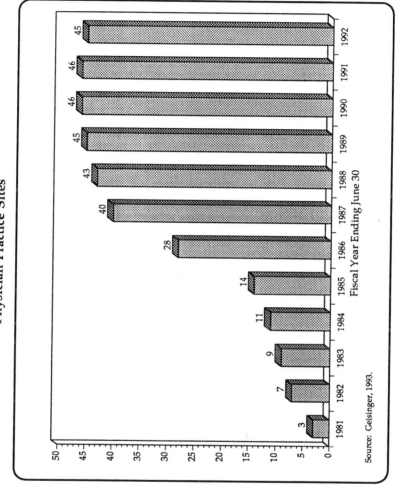

EXHIBIT E.
Growth in the Number of Geisinger Clinic
Physician Practice Sites

Fiscal Year Ending June 30

Source: Geisinger, 1993.

EXHIBIT F.
Geisinger System Corporate Structure

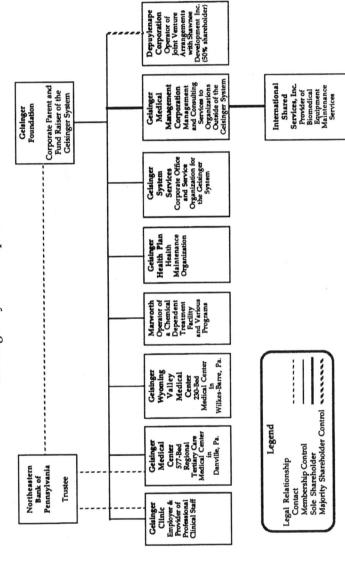

Source: Geisinger Sytem, 1992.

duplication of functions, and that the decision-making process needed to be improved. As one example, a separate financial organization had been established for the clinic. Both the clinic and hospital had human resources departments. Therefore, in December, 1992, the organization was restructured along geographic lines with three regions. All functions within each region were consolidated into one organization headed by a team consisting of a senior vice president for operations and a physician-leader. (This was the typical pattern of management at Geisinger — physician-leaders paired with trained and experienced administrators.)

In 1993 the Central Region accounted for 65 percent of Geisinger's physicians and 74 percent of its employees. The Eastern Region accounted for 21 percent of the physicians and employees. The more sparsely populated Western Region represented 14 percent of Geisinger's physicians and five percent of the system's workforce.

Jack Hartman, Senior Vice President for Legal Services, said that there were several reasons for retaining the 1981 legal structure. "We balanced the pros and cons of keeping the structure versus getting rid of all the corporations. The bottom line was that we decided to keep the structure." He also said that the new organizational structure was intended to eliminate the "vertical silos." "We wanted to enhance teamwork and break down barriers."

Under the new structure, the Geisinger Foundation board and its executive committee were pivotal. Thirteen of the 14 members were business and community leaders (including one non-Geisinger physician) from the service area; Dr. Heydt, Geisinger's CEO, was the fourteenth member.

Members of the executive committee of the foundation served as board members for the corporations remaining from the 1981 reorganization (e.g., medical center, clinic, health plan).

The December, 1992, organizational chart is attached as Exhibit G.

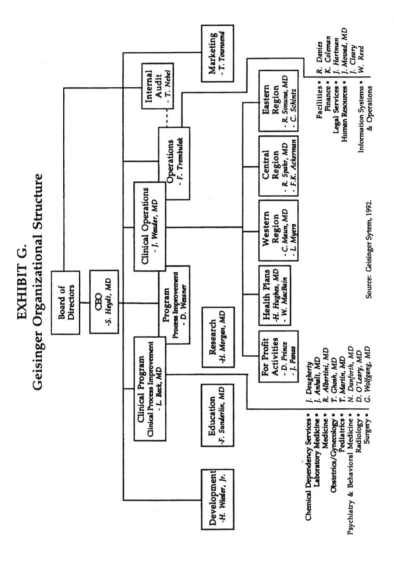

EXHIBIT G.
Geisinger Organizational Structure

Source: Geisinger Sytem, 1992.

Geisinger Health Plan (GHP)

Early history of GHP. The Geisinger Health Plan was established in 1972 as part of the HMO initiative of the Nixon Administration; Dr. Paul Ellwood was instrumental in implementing this federal program. Geisinger was one of six health care organizations that received an HEW grant to organize an HMO; this was viewed as a pilot project. Federal funding was slightly in excess of $500,000.

Blue Cross was a partner in the HMO, and was responsible for the actuarial studies and marketing. The service area covered five counties, although the plan was limited to residents of Danville and Montour County. Ackerman said, "We deliberately kept the HMO low key. We didn't want to upset physicians who were referring to Geisinger specialists. In fact, by 1985 we had only 12,000 participants, and two-thirds of them were Geisinger employees and their families."

The 1985 changes. In the mid-1980s, Geisinger made a decision to more aggressively market the health plan. Blue Cross was separated from the venture, and Geisinger hired marketing and management personnel and a medical director.

According to Robert Spahr, MD, Senior Vice President for Clinical Operations in the Central Region, Geisinger's leaders anticipated continued erosion in reimbursement from Medicare and private payors. "We wanted more control over our destiny, and we saw an expanded HMO as a big part of the answer."

Howard Hughes, MD, who was in charge of GHP in 1993, was trained in emergency medicine and had become involved in various management activities since joining Geisinger in 1977. When the decision was made to place more emphasis on the health plan, he became Medical Director and then Senior Vice President (prior to the 1992 reorganization, he was president of the health plan).

Growth in GHP. In commenting on the financial performance of the plan, Dr. Hughes said that revenues in the fiscal year ending June 30, 1992, were $116 million. Operating profits were $2.1 million. He said that the plan reached break-even in 1988.

Exhibit H shows the growth in health plan membership from 1985 through June 1993. As noted, GHP has grown rapidly, reaching 52,000

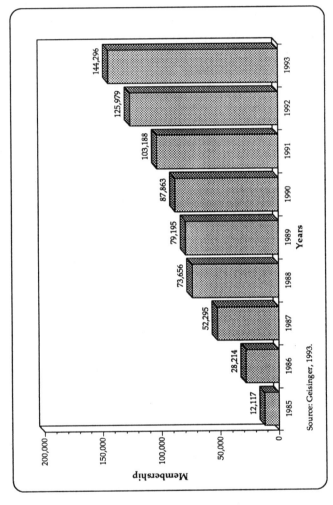

EXHIBIT H.
Geisinger Health Plan,
Membership Growth @ June 30,
Fiscal Years 1985-1993

Source: Geisinger, 1993.

members in 1987, two years after the decision to promote participation more aggressively.

Premium rate increases have averaged 8.6 percent annually since 1985. And, according to Dr. Hughes, "We started at a low base, probably too low." As a result of these below-average rate increases, the GHP was competitively priced within the service area. A New York Times article said that GHP was the lowest cost HMO in Pennsylvania (*The New York Times*, March 18, 1993).

In terms of the secrets of success in managing the health plan, Dr. Hughes said that it came down to physician utilization. He said that 90 to 95 percent of the GHP subscriber encounters were with Geisinger physicians (there were 350 non-Geisinger doctors on the panel), and that the Geisinger doctors were learning how to practice effectively in a capitated environment. "We don't have to police them or look over their shoulders. This helps keep our administrative costs down." (On this point, he noted that the HMO had a staff of 123, or about half of the staff of a normal HMO with equivalent membership.)

Dr. Hughes noted that one of the key factors in expanding health plan membership in the past has been the number of primary care locations. In addition, he said, "The Geisinger name has also been a powerful marketing force." Looking ahead, Dr. Hughes said that in order to expand the size of the HMO, Geisinger would need to add several more primary care practice sites, and that the health plan had already identified where some of these sites should be located.

The future. Growth in GHP was a major component of Geisinger's strategic plan in 1993. David Wessner, Executive Vice President, Program and Process Improvement, said that Geisinger had no choice but to expand the coverage of its health plan. He said, "We need to have around 600,000 members. If we don't have one-third of the market, we aren't a player with the consolidation that we expect to take place."

He went on, "What will it take to grow our HMO enrollment fast enough? We have to add more primary care locations and increase the size of several that already exist. We have to make primary care more efficient. We have to develop new insurance products, such as a Medicare-risk product. We have to work with other physicians and hospitals in the region; we can't do it all with our own system."

Frank Trembulak said that Geisinger as a system continued to be provider-dominated. "We need to increase the size of the financing mechanism in order to achieve a better balance. I believe that when GHP represents 40 percent of our business (it was around 20 percent in 1993), we will be a significantly different and more cost-effective organization."

Dr. Heydt agreed and said that if Geisinger was to become more efficient, a higher proportion of its patients had to come from HMOs or other risk contracts. "It would help us to have more of our patients in GHP. We would also like to see Medicare set up a risk contract so we could gain experience in handling older patients on a capitated basis. The way it is now we are a schizophrenic organization with a mix of capitation and fee-for-service."

Other opportunities for expansion of membership in the GHP included the small business market and Medicare. "We are seriously evaluating the possibility of a competitive health plan — the Medicare risk contract. We think we know enough about running an HMO that we could do well with the Medicare population."

In discussing the amount of start-up capital needed for an HMO, Dr. Hughes said that there were too many variables to formulate a hard and fast rule. "However, I wouldn't want to do it without having $4 million to $5 million available."

Physician Compensation

Geisinger had two different compensation methods — one for physicians at the main campus and a different one for doctors at the 43 other sites. Physicians in locations away from Danville were paid based on productivity; the system for these doctors was traditional. Since many of the physicians in Danville were performing research, teaching, in administration and performing activities other than direct patient care, determining compensation was more complex.

Kenneth Ackerman noted that, until the early 1980s, all physicians were on salary. "They weren't all paid the same; the compensation system reflected supply and demand. However, they were not paid based on the dollars they brought into the system." This changed when Geisinger began to expand its network, and paid primary care physicians who came into the system on a different basis. "They were accustomed to having their compensation based on productivity, and we attempted to maintain this type of system for this group of doctors."

According to Dr. Heydt, Geisinger had a relatively narrow compensation range. In other words, many specialists earned less than they could in private practice, and primary care physicians earned more. Primary care physicians earned $90,000 to $120,000, and specialists earned as much as $375,000.

One surgeon who generated more than $1.5 million in annual billings said he earned less than the $375,000 earned by the cardiovascular surgeon. "I know I could earn more in private practice but that's not why I came here. I believe in group practice, and enjoy participating in the education and research here at Geisinger."

Other Aspects of Geisinger

Corporate culture. The founding physicians, and others who played a key role in the formation and subsequent development of the organization, are honored and revered. Buildings are named after Drs. Foss and Bush (the founder and his successor); the primary care outpatient center is named after a beloved nursing manager and leader, Emma Jean Knapper, who devoted 40 years to Geisinger. Pictures and paintings of the founders and physician leaders, and key events in the history of the organization (ground breakings, grand openings of new wings) are prominently displayed in the hallways of the clinics and hospitals. Geisinger distributes two books written by Dr. Foss.

Dr. Spahr said that the history of Geisinger has had a major impact on its corporate culture. "We have attracted people who agree with what we are trying to accomplish and the way we do things. On the down-side, our system won't tolerate outliers — individuals who chafe under the constraints of our culture. We encourage them to leave. Fortunately, this doesn't happen very often."

Dr. Heydt said that the Geisinger corporate culture was part of its competitive advantage. "We have a common value system. We can conduct planning together and agree on what we want to accomplish."

O. Fred Miller, MD, Director of the Dermatology Department, said that being at Geisinger, and working with residents, keeps him up to date with new developments in his field. "For example, we have a journal club that meets every Wednesday morning for one and a half hours to review articles in our two journals. One of the dermatologists gets up at 4 AM to prepare; we take it seriously. I know I wouldn't be challenged to do this if I were in private practice."

There was disagreement among Geisinger physicians about the importance of physician administrators continuing to practice medicine. Dr. Heydt, an oral and maxillofacial surgeon and President of the Geisinger Foundation, dropped his medical practice several years ago. "This is a big job. The board pays me to be CEO, not to practice medicine. Also, I don't have time to keep up with my field, and I am concerned that the quality of care I could deliver to patients would not be as high as I would like it to be."

At the same time, several other physician-administrators at Geisinger practice medicine 10 to 20 percent of the time. The head of the health plan, who is board-certified in emergency medicine, said that if he had to give up practicing medicine as a condition of being an administrator, he would not take the administrative job.

Other physician-administrators at Geisinger said that they enjoyed practicing medicine and believed it was part of maintaining their credibility with other doctors. One physician said, "When we take off our white coats, physicians do not view us as doctors; we become administrators. This has always been a physician-driven organization, and I hate to see that change." He went on to say that he has been accused of having a "shop-foreman mentality."

Teaching and research. The research and education programs at Geisinger are an important component of the health system. In 1992, $8 million was spent on research with two-thirds of this amount coming from Geisinger. The remaining one-third was funded by grants and gifts.

Geisinger has had a long-term graduate medical education program, with 200 residents and fellows in training in 1993. Demand for residencies was high, with several department chairmen reporting more than 100 applications for each opening.

Information systems. William Reed, Senior Vice President, Operations/Geisinger System and Chief Information Officer, said that all of Geisinger's information systems are centralized. "All systems are common, meaning that lab, pharmacy and other applications are run on the same system. There are very few stand-alone applications."

Reed said that the strength of Geisinger's information systems was in the financial areas. The clinical information system was more limited. "A new system is in the works that will include a clinical repository for reports and a new patient order system." Changes in the information system are designed to ensure that patients receive the same standard of care throughout the system. Reed said that Geisinger was attempting to consolidate everything being done for a patient, with the goal of attaining system-wide continuity of care.

Kenneth Ackerman said, "Defined, standardized clinical protocols and outcome indicators are being developed for system-wide use. Physicians will be better equipped to monitor performance and, as a result, take corrective action when necessary."

Geisinger had 115 employees on the staff of its information system department, with half involved in programming, development and enhancements. The annual budget for information systems was $14 million.

Quality initiatives and outcomes measurement. Dr. Laurence Beck and David Wessner team up to head the quality improvement initiative at Geisinger. According to Dr. Beck, Geisinger has trained most of its managers and has several teams working. "We have been impressed with what Proctor & Gamble has accomplished. The company has a 3,000-employee paper plant in our area and their staff has been working with us. We have probably learned more from them than from anyone else." He said that six teams were working on clinical guidelines, and that there were a large number of less formal teams at work.

In terms of outcomes measurement, Dr. Beck said that Geisinger was not as far along. "However, it is part of the responsibility of each formal quality improvement team to develop measurable outcomes. Other than that, we are part of MedisGroups. We stack up OK." He noted that Geisinger also has a federally-funded project related to medical outcomes.

David Wessner said that the payoffs Geisinger expected from its continuous quality improvement program would include customer loyalty, lower costs, employee buy-in, and superior quality. He added, "The content of our quality of care may be high, perhaps tops in the region. But, I am not sure our service delivery is nearly as good as it could be. We have to work harder to differentiate Geisinger from other providers."

Geisinger systematically measured patient satisfaction through the use of surveys. Response rates were sufficiently large to evaluate the performance of each of the network sites. Theodore Townsend, Senior Vice President for Marketing Operations, said that 70 percent of the patients rated the performance of Geisinger physicians as excellent. "However, this doesn't mean we are satisfied." David Wessner said that in his opir'on, surveys of customer satisfaction were more valuable than financial information systems. "We haven't been giving these types of surveys enougʰ attention."

Malpractice insurance. Geisinger provided two types of malpractice coverage to augment the Pennsylvania program. Keith Coleman said that the combination of the favorable experience of Geisinger physicians and the ability of the organization to use its size to negotiate favorable rates has saved Geisinger several million dollars since 1982.

Major Accomplishments/Lessons Learned

Frank Trembulak said that Geisinger's two major accomplishments over the past 15 years have been the development of its primary care network and the success of its health plan. "These two strategies are the underpinnings of the future of Geisinger."

Trembulak said that one of the lessons learned at Geisinger is that the problems it faces are not that much different from those faced by other organizations. "Physicians and hospitals in traditional settings have trouble attracting and retaining primary care doctors, and their specialists are tense about the future of health care and how it will affect them. We have these same problems. We are concerned about maintaining adequate payment sources; so are other providers."

Another lesson learned from the experience of Geisinger is the importance of being open to change. Trembulak said, "You can't come to the table with a fixed agenda; it won't work. One of the questions that should be asked is: 'What is the best use of the resources we have available?' We should also be asking about what can be done to better identify and meet community needs. This is not the time to dig in." He went on to say that Geisinger has learned that it has to continually ask what can be done to produce cost-effective care. "Other organizations need to confront this issue also."

Dr. Hughes believes that when physicians buy into the managed care philosophy, an HMO will be successful. "I can tell when the light goes on with our own physicians. It is a new way of looking at the practice of medicine. They begin to come up with ideas of how to save money and provide better treatment, and they get excited about it."

Issues for the Future

Dr. Heydt said, "Our fundamental challenge is to care for more people at less cost. We don't have any choice with the growth in managed care, especially capitated systems and health care reform."

Another issue of concern to Dr. Heydt and many others was the sizing of the organization. "Will capitation force us to size Geisinger differently? We believe it will, and we are studying the matter now. This is a very sensitive issue."

Frank Trembulak said that Geisinger needed to become more cost effective. "We need to utilize our resources better. We should consider extending the hours of some of our facilities. There have to be ways we can use our capital assets more effectively." He went on. "We have to change our mentality and realize that we can't control our revenues. However, we can control our costs."

Dr. Spahr said that he was concerned about managing specialty services. "Even though we are emphasizing primary care, these physicians may not always be the low-cost providers. I know from my own experience that a pulmonologist may make more effective use of hospital resources for his or her patients; therefore, having a specialist treat lung problems may be a better way to go."

He was also concerned about changes in the competitive environment and believed that independent primary care physicians in the service area would increasingly be called on to make choices about which systems they would be part of. "Even though many of them refer to us now, will we be their choice in the future?"

Looking ahead, Kenneth Ackerman said that Geisinger needs to continue to function more like a "seamless" health care system.

Jack Hartman, Senior Vice President for Legal Services, said that he is concerned that Geisinger is being asked to carry a disproportionate share of patients on Medicaid, Medicare or without insurance. "Other physicians and hospitals in our service area are clearly shifting their poor-paying patients to Geisinger."

Dr. Laurence Beck expressed concern that financial pressures would drive Geisinger away from medical research and teaching.

Theodore Townsend said that he is concerned about Geisinger's ability to maintain its differentiation. "Our history, large concentration of specialists, and reputation for quality were important differentiating factors in the past. But, as other physician groups and hospitals in our service area integrate, we could lose some of our advantages. Also, some of the competing health plans are likely to establish strong relationships with other medical groups and compete with the Geisinger Health Plan. We have our work cut out for us."

---

* We appreciated the efforts of F. Kenneth Ackerman, Jr., Senior Vice President for Operations, Geisinger's Central Region, in arranging the interviews and providing the background information required to complete this case study.

Case Study #9

KAISER PERMANENTE/
SAINT JOSEPH HOSPITAL
Denver, Colorado

— **Persons Interviewed** —

Sister Marianna Bauder, President, Saint Joseph Hospital
Chris Binkley, Senior Vice President and Regional Manager,
    Kaiser Permanente
Jon Boline, MD, Chairman, Medwest Board
Ben Chao, Information Services Director, Kaiser Permanente
David Charles, MD, Chief of Staff, Saint Joseph Hospital
Toby Cole, MD, President, Colorado Permanente Medical Group
Robert Collins, Chairman, Saint Joseph Hospital Board
Greg Ippen, MD, Medwest Physician
Bill Reimers, MD, Former Medical Director and Founding Physician
Bev Schulman, Vice President, Planning and Marketing,
    Saint Joseph Hospital
LeRoy Sides, MD, Director of Key Care
Steven Tomme, Vice President and Regional Marketing Manager,
    Kaiser Permanente
Scott Waldrop, Vice President, Information Services, Saint Joseph Hospital
Dennis Wilson, Chief Financial Officer, Saint Joseph Hospital
Sanford Zisman, Board Member, Saint Joseph Hospital

July, 1993

EXHIBIT A.
Colorado and Denver Metropolitan Area

KAISER PERMANENTE/
SAINT JOSEPH HOSPITAL
Denver, Colorado

Kaiser Permanente, a national group-model HMO, had 280,000 health plan members in the Denver Metropolitan Area in mid-1993. The Colorado Permanente Medical Group, which provides medical services for health plan members, had 430 physicians. Kaiser Permanente's Colorado Region generated $430 million in revenues in 1992.

Kaiser Permanente Health Plan contracted with Saint Joseph Hospital for most of its inpatient care and for many other hospital-based services. Kaiser Permanente (KP) patients represented an average of 55 percent of the inpatient days of Saint Joseph Hospital; this percentage has grown over the years that the two organizations have had a contractual relationship but remained constant from 1991 through mid-1993.

In addition, Saint Joseph Hospital's medical staff included another 500 private practice physicians. The hospital had developed a number of physician-hospital organizations and integrated approaches.

Exhibit A is a map showing the location of Denver in Colorado. Saint Joseph Hospital is approximately one-half mile east of the central business district, in what is generally considered to be the hospital district of Denver.

The Denver Area Health Care Marketplace

Kaiser Permanente and Saint Joseph Hospital (SJH) operated in an environment characterized by heavy managed care market penetration, intense competition among acute care hospitals and a surplus of physicians, especially specialists.

Demographics of the Denver Area. The Denver Area had a 1993 population of 2.0 million. After experiencing an economic slump from 1984 through 1989, the Denver Area economy had resumed its long-term pattern of employment and economic growth.

The Denver Area population was younger than average, with 10 percent of the residents in Medicare, compared with over 13 percent nationally.

Health plan coverage patterns. Exhibit B shows the growth in membership in Kaiser Permanente and other Denver Area HMOs over the 1986 through 1992 period. The merger of Comprecare and TakeCare occurred in 1993.

Exhibit B.

HMO Enrollment in the Denver Metro Area, 1986 and 1992 (January 1, Each Year)

HMO	1986		1992	
	Number	Percent	Number	Percent
1. Kaiser Permanente	160,000	49.2%	268,000	44.0%
2. Comprecare	100,000	30.8	140,000	23.0
3. MetLife	600	0.2	59,000	9.7
4. HMO Colorado	32,000	9.8	41,000	6.7
5. TakeCare*	6,000	1.8	38,000	6.2
6. CIGNA	600	0.2	34,000	5.6
7. All Others**	26,000	8.0	28,500	4.7
Total	325,200	100.0%	608,500	100.0%
HMO Enrollment - Denver Metro Population		18.6%		33.8%

*   Formerly Lincoln National.
** Includes Aetna, Exclusive Health Care, Humana Health Care Plan, PruCare, Qual-Med, and Rocky Mountain HMO.
Source: HealthCare Computer Corporation of America.

Acute care hospitals. In 1993 there were 17 acute care hospitals in the Denver Area representing 5,805 licensed beds. The average occupancy rate in 1992 was 57.5 percent based on available beds.

Saint Joseph Hospital's major competitors were Presbyterian/St. Luke's Medical Center (a new 676-bed facility), located right across the street from SJH, Rose Medical Center, Provenant Health Partners (St. Anthony Hospital Central), Porter Memorial Hospital and several other hospitals.

At the time of the case study, Swedish Medical Center, located on the south side of the Denver Area, and the P/SL Healthcare System (downtown hospital plus Aurora Presbyterian Hospital and the Centennial Healthcare Plaza outpatient center in southeast Denver) had announced their intention to merge.

The Healthcare Initiative (THI). Along with Rose, Swedish and Lutheran Medical Centers, Saint Joseph Hospital and its private practice physicians were participants in THI, the joint managed care initiative of the three hospitals. In 1993, THI had 40,000 lives covered, and was willing to take on risk contracting. However, the Swedish-P/SL merger proved to be disruptive to the THI group, since P/SL was a major competitor of both Rose and Saint Joseph Hospital; Swedish was dropped as of mid-1993.

Presence of large clinics and integrated systems. The Denver health care marketplace was fragmented in terms of medical group practices. Accord Medical Centers, a multispecialty clinic located in southeast Denver, about two to three miles from Saint Joseph Hospital, was the largest in the metro area with 45 physicians.

The combination of Kaiser Permanente and Saint Joseph Hospital represented the most highly integrated health care system in the Denver Area. Several other physician groups and hospitals had developed physician-hospital organizations. For example, Rose Medical Center and a group of 45 primary care physicians had formed the Premier Medical Group, a clinic without walls. However, in most cases the number of physicians involved in these organizations was small relative to the size of the medical staffs of the hospitals. None of the hospitals owned a health plan.

The History and Growth of Kaiser Permanente in Colorado

The Kaiser Permanente Colorado Region was one of 12 in the United States. Nationally, Kaiser Permanente (KP) had over 6.6 million members as of year end 1992; over two-thirds of these were in California. KP employed over 9,000 physicians and had 236 medical offices. Its 1992 revenues were $11.0 billion. The system also owned 7,772 licensed acute care beds (Kaiser Permanente, *1992 Annual Report*, page 22).

Early history of KP in Colorado. Kaiser Permanente came to Colorado in 1969, and it has had a contractual relationship with Saint Joseph Hospital since the early days. Kaiser Permanente's Colorado and Cleveland Regions were the first established outside the West Coast. The

Northern California Region sponsored Cleveland and the Southern California Region sponsored the Colorado start up.

The first physician, Bill Reimers, MD, a general surgeon, was on the medical staff of Saint Joseph Hospital at the time. He had been in private practice for 16 years prior to joining KP. Although in the beginning, Dr. Reimers maintained his private practice, he noted that referrals from other private practice physicians dropped off dramatically. He said, "Several of my colleagues told me that our Permanente Group staff was excellent, but that they disagreed with the approach. Some of them thought we were involved in socialized medicine."

Dr. Toby Cole, an internist and president of the Colorado Permanente Medical Group, joined CPMG in 1971. In discussing the relationship with Saint Joseph Hospital, he said, "Before I could be credentialed at Saint Joseph, I had to attend multiple meetings. Private practice physicians got in the first time. Some of the physicians there thought we were socialists at best."

Growth in membership. Exhibit C shows the trend in membership in Kaiser Permanente since its establishment. As of spring, 1993, this health plan had 280,000 members, representing 15 percent of the Denver Area health care market. KP exceeded its breakeven point during the 1974-75 period when enrollment reached 60,000 members.

Steven Tomme, Vice President and Regional Marketing Manager, noted that in the early 1980s KP was a low profile organization. "We did not advertise. In fact, I was the director of enrollment. We didn't think in terms of marketing."

He pointed out that one of the reasons for the surge in growth in enrollment in the late 1980s was that KP did not have a rate increase in 1987 and 1988 and had a modest increase in 1989. This was during a period when competing health plans had large rate increases. "As a result, we grew so fast we had to cut off enrollment. We couldn't hire physicians fast enough to keep up."

Tomme said that KP initially positioned itself as the alternative to Blue Cross and Blue Shield of Colorado which was then only in indemnity insurance. "Our pitch to employers was to offer their employees a dual choice, and since we were cheaper, it wouldn't cost them anything." He noted, "Now with the growth of our organization and managed care, we are viewed by many as the market leader. Our competitors now position themselves as alternatives to Kaiser."

Exhibit C.

**Growth in Kaiser Permanente Membership in Colorado,
1969 through 1993**

Year	Membership Growth Total	Increase
1969	2,808	2,808
1970	13,491	10,683
1971	23,327	9,836
1972	40,256	16,929
1973	50,144	9,888
1974	59,813	9,669
1975	64,968	5,155
1976	75,952	10,984
1977	90,528	14,576
1978	101,978	11,450
1979	108,484	6,506
1980	116,121	7,637
1981	124,238	8,117
1982	135,410	11,160
1983	147,590	12,180
1984	157,346	9,756
1985	161,240	3,894
1986	163,754	2,514
1987	173,101	9,347
1988	195,190	22,089
1989	227,674	32,484
1990	246,706	19,032
1991	264,192	17,486
1992	275,536*	11,334*
1993	285,770*	10,234*

* Projected year end 1992 & 1993
Source: Kaiser Permanente, July, 1993.

Establishment of medical group offices. Kaiser Permanente has followed the practice of investing in its own medical offices located throughout the Denver Area. These facilities are usually 24,000 square feet to start, and provide space for 12 to 20 physicians with emphasis on primary care in all locations except Franklin Street. Exhibit D shows the locations of the Kaiser Permanente's 13 medical offices in the Denver Area.

EXHIBIT D.
Kaiser Permanente Medical Office Locations, 1993

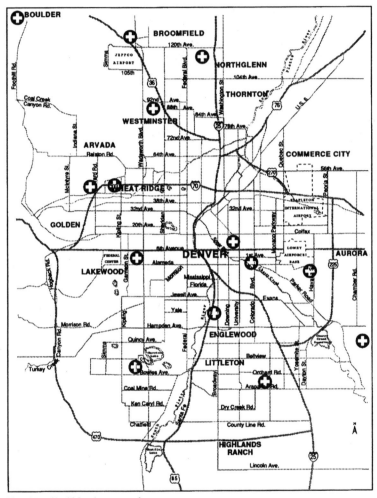

Note: Mental health locations are not shown.
Source: Kaiser Permanente, June 1993.

KP began with two medical offices, one on Franklin Street adjacent to Saint Joseph Hospital, and one in Lakewood, a western suburb of the Denver Area. These offices are normally planned to handle five-year's of growth. Dr. Cole said that in identifying the first two suburban offices — Lakewood and Thornton — KP relied on the services of a demographer, and over the initial years established offices in each quadrant (west, north, south and east) of the urban area. Additional offices were added to take the pressure off the initial four locations and the Franklin Street office.

In terms of planning for new locations for medical offices, Chris Binkley, Senior Vice President and Regional Manager of the Kaiser Foundation Health Plan of Colorado, said that KP tries to minimize a member's driving time to 10 to 15 minutes. This usually translates into each office serving enrollees living within a four-mile radius.

In terms of new medical offices, Binkley said that the 15-year facility plan anticipated four new medical offices in the Denver Area over the next five years.

Growth of the Colorado Permanente Medical Group. Dr. Cole said that the original physicians joined the group because they were pioneers. "They liked the concept. Some of them came out of the military, and they appreciated the benefits of a group practice without the limitations of the military. They certainly didn't come with us because of the pay."

According to Dr. Cole, primary care physicians were added as membership increased. "You can generally figure that for each 765 members we will add a physician. On average, across all Kaiser Permanente facilities, each doctor requires 4.6 persons as support staff. All of this is a function of membership." Therefore, CPMG's growth has paralleled that of enrollment in the health plan. As noted earlier, CPMG had 430 physicians in early 1993 with approximately 50 percent in primary care. (One of the objectives of KP was to increase the proportion of primary care physicians to 60 percent of the total.) Exhibit E shows the growth in the number of physicians from 1983 to 1992.

Exhibit E.

Growth in Number of Physicians,
Colorado Permanente Medical Group, 1983 - 1992

Year	Full-Time Physicians	Part-Time Physicians
1983	135	6
1984	151	4
1985	169	4
1986	177	7
1987	195	12
1988	216	14
1989	271	18
1990	324	21
1991	339	22
1992	394	37

Source: Kaiser Permanente, July, 1993.

According to Dr. Cole, the CPMG receives 27 percent of the revenue coming into KP for the provision of physician services. "This is our annual budget, and we work within it."

Governance and management. The CPMG is governed by six physicians and Dr. Cole. Physician board members are elected by the shareholders (to be a shareholder, a physician had to be employed at KP for a minimum of three years and be accepted by the other shareholders).

Kaiser Permanente has a long-standing policy of pairing physicians and administrators to perform management roles in the organization. Dr. Cole said, "While this helps our physicians get comfortable with management positions, we expect them to improve in their management skills. They have shown that they can do it."

Hospital ownership versus contracting. KP began planning for its own hospital in 1980. A site had been selected, plans drawn and construction contracts awarded. The ownership of its own acute care facility would have been consistent with KP's practice in other regions. According to Dr. Cole, "We had $2.5 million invested in planning before we reached the point of re-evaluating the advantages and disadvantages of building our own facility."

He went on, "In the 1970s, hospital capacity in the Denver Area was pushed to the limit. It wasn't until the early 1980s that there was a recognition that the metro area may have too many acute care beds. This caused us to re-think our strategy of building and owning a hospital."

In 1985, Kaiser Permanente and Saint Joseph Hospital re-negotiated their relationship, and KP management decided that it would be more cost effective and responsible to contract with an established hospital rather than building a new one.

Binkley said that the construction of the new hospital would have required a $60 to $80 million capital investment. "We began to analyze the alternative uses for these funds, and realized that we could build five primary care offices for what it cost to build a hospital; that is what we did. In retrospect, that decision helped us grow by enabling us to move more quickly in establishing medical offices in locations convenient to present and prospective subscribers." He went on, "This was not an easy decision. Some of our advisors thought that it was essential that we own our own hospital."

Kaiser Permanente's use of other hospitals. Saint Joseph Hospital received about 80 percent of KP's inpatient admissions. The remaining 20 percent went to P/SL for mental health services, Children's Hospital for certain pediatric cases and to Boulder Community Hospital for KP enrollees in Boulder and Longmont. (These two communities are part of the Denver Metro Area, but are 35 miles from Saint Joseph Hospital.) KP also contracted for emergency services at two other metro area hospitals.

Physician compensation. Dr. Cole said, "We hire physicians at comparable rates to those in the community. This may place us above the average for certain doctors, but overall we are not that much different. Salaries increase automatically for six years." Dr. Cole said that in a good year there is a four to five percent bonus paid to physicians. "In an excellent year, it might run a percent or two above that, but this does not represent a significant proportion of yearly income."

He pointed out that the range between an established primary care physician and a specialist may be 2.5 times. "We consider this to be a rather narrow range, at least compared with the ratio of incomes of private practice specialists to primary care doctors."

Recruiting and retaining physicians. Dr. Cole said that physicians typically join the CPMG for a combination of reasons that include "not having to compete for patients, job security, and a desire for a more orderly life style. We receive 15 applications for each opening. Right now internists are the most difficult to recruit."

The turnover rate among physicians was low, between three and five percent per year. Dr. Cole said that what pleased him was that when physicians left, it was for the right reasons -- a desire for additional training, interest in moving to a different part of the country. The average tenure of a CPMG physician exceeded eight years.

Saint Joseph Hospital

Early history. Established in 1873 by four members of the Sisters of Charity of Leavenworth, Saint Joseph Hospital was the first private hospital in Colorado. The hospital was originally known as Saint Vincents. In 1899, the "Unsinkable Molly Brown" threw a party to raise money for the hospital. The present 565-bed facility, the largest in the state, was opened in 1964.

The past five years. Exhibit F summarizes a number of key indicators for SJH for the 1989 through 1993 period. Over this period of time, inpatient utilization has decreased from 124,000 inpatient days in 1989 to 122,000 days in 1993; this was less of a drop than that experienced by all hospitals in the Denver Area for this time period.

Exhibit G summarizes the financial performance of SJH over this same five-year period. The hospital's net operating revenues have increased from $111.9 million in fiscal year 1989 to $166.1 million in 1993. Revenue over expenses was $9.3 million in 1993; this compared with $6.4 million in 1989.

Exhibit F.
Trend in Selected Statistics, Saint Joseph Hospital,
1988 Through 1992 (Fiscal Years ending May 31)

	1989	1990	1991	1992	1993
Patient Days	124,354	123,490	118,843	119,947	121,977
Admissions	23,722	23,639	24,568	25,367	25,621
Outpatient Visits	145,327	160,121	187,940	204,552	221,064
Deliveries	5,144	5,297	5,282	5,606	5,117
Length of Stay	5.2	5.2	4.8	4.7	4.8
Surgery Hours	33,754	34,384	38,559	40,270	38,756

Source: Saint Joseph Hospital Trend of Selected Statistics, June, 1993.

Exhibit G.
Saint Joseph Hospital, Financial Performance,
1988 Through 1992 (in thousands)

	1989	1990	1991	1992	1993
Net Operating Revenue	$111,987	$120,520	$136,847	$154,620	$166,149
Revenue Over Expenses	6,419	4,406	1,512	9,025	9,284
Assets	127,817	132,228	133,419	142,673	154,817
Liabilities	22,432	21,787	21,268	22,081	25,666
Fund Balance	105,385	110,441	112,151	120,592	129,150

Source: Saint Joseph Hospital, Statements of Revenue and Expenses for years ended May 31 each year; Saint Joseph Hospital Balance Sheets, May 31, each year.

At the end of fiscal year 1993, Saint Joseph Hospital had assets of $154.8 million and total long-term debt of less than $1 million. Current liabilities were $25.7 million.

Saint Joseph Hospital performed more open heart surgeries, 450 per year, than any hospital in the state. More babies were born at SJH (over 5,000 per year) than in any other hospital in Colorado.

Hospital leadership and organization.   Sister Marianna Bauder became CEO of SJH in November, 1990, after five years as CEO of St. Mary's Hospital in Grand Junction, Colorado. In addition to degrees in chemistry and biology, she has an MBA degree from Notre Dame.

The hospital's board consisted of 13 members — seven from the Sisters of Charity of Leavenworth, and six from the community. The entire board meets quarterly and the local board meets eight times a year. The hospital's organizational chart is shown on Exhibit H.

The Chairman of the Board of Trustees, Robert Collins, was the founder of Cobe Laboratories, a large medical supply firm.

The impact of Kaiser Permanente. The impact of Kaiser Permanente on SJH has been increasing since 1969. According to Dennis Wilson, CFO, KP accounted for approximately 15,000 of the hospital's 25,000 annual admissions. However, since KP's average length of stay was less, the health plan represented about 55 percent of inpatient utilization of the Saint Joseph facility.

Wilson noted that the impact of KP increased beginning on January 1, 1986, when the health plan entered into the Medicare risk contracting business. This portion of KP's business increased from approximately 10,000 lives to 25,000 in 1993. Wilson said that these 25,000 Medicare patients accounted for 40 percent of the revenues Saint Joseph received from KP.

Wilson also said that the KP contract does not call for Kaiser Permanente to pay for hospital beds "at the margin." He said, "They are too big to buy on the margin. This might work for a small health plan, but not for Kaiser." He noted that Kaiser Permanente has been fair in its dealings with Saint Joseph.

The contract was set up with a five-year roll over. In other words, rates and other elements of the contract were negotiated annually, but for future years. For example, the 1993 round of negotiations solidified rates and other aspects of the contract through 1995.

The strategy of cultivating both KP and private physicians. Sister Marianna Bauder said that Saint Joseph Hospital intended to continue to maintain its private practice base, and that the hospital has several different initiatives to make sure that various physician groups succeed in the future. The relationships between SJH and Medwest, Key Care, and the Accord Medical Center are described later in this case study.

EXHIBIT H.
Saint Joseph Hospital Organizational Chart

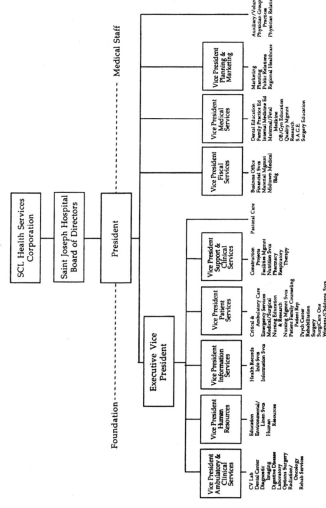

Source: Saint Joseph Hospital, June 1993.

Physician leadership trends. Robert Collins, the Chairman of the Board of Trustees, noted that there was one physician (Jon Boline, MD) on the hospital's board, and that the chief of the medical staff (David Charles, MD) also met with the board. Collins also noted that the hospital has had a full-time vice president for medical affairs for the past six years. "These are two aspects of our recognition of the importance of physicians to this organization."

Low-cost provider status of SJH. Saint Joseph Hospital was recognized as the low-cost provider among Denver Area hospitals. Independent data collected and reported by the Colorado Health Data Commission and the Colorado Hospital Association supported this contention.

Why was Saint Joseph so much more cost effective than other Denver Area hospitals? According to Sanford Zisman, Vice Chairman of the SJH Board, there were three reasons:

- *Lack of debt and interest payments.* "This alone gives us a 10 to 15 percent advantage of more highly leveraged hospitals."

- *The Kaiser Permanente contract.* "This gives Saint Joseph Hospital the ability to spread its fixed costs over a larger base and to operate more efficiently."

- *Quality of care.* "It is generally true for hospitals that it is more cost effective to do things right the first time."

Dennis Wilson, CFO, attributed Saint Joseph Hospital's economic advantages to a multitude of factors, including the volume of patients from Kaiser Permanente, cost-effective practice patterns by Permanente physicians and others, lack of debt and low average length of stay. "We have been focusing on efficiency for 15 years; we have never played the game of raising our rates to what the market would bear. Consequently, we have low overhead, and a large volume of patients to absorb the overhead expenses we do have."

On the matter of why Saint Joseph was the low-cost hospital in the community, Robert Collins said that he believes it was due primarily to four factors:

(1) Lack of debt and therefore, lack of funds needed for debt service. "This alone can make our costs 10 percent lower than those of our competitors."

(2)   Favorable ratio of employees per discharge.

(3)   Better use of inpatient capacity; higher occupancy rates.

(4)   Less spending on marketing and promotional activities.

Quality of care. Sister Marianna Bauder said that SJH was one of 550 hospitals participating in the MedisGroups' MediQual programs, and had been involved for seven years. She said that the hospital was ranked fourth out of the 100 hospitals that perform open heart surgery and was in the top 10 in measurements of quality of care for pneumonia, stroke, myocardial infarction (heart attack) and congestive heart failure. "We have always ranked well above the norm in all clinical areas."

She said there were several reasons for the hospital's ability to achieve quality. One factor was the number of long-term employees; 350 had been with the hospital for 15 years or more. Volume of patients and procedures was another reason; SJH and its cardiovascular surgeons performed more by-pass surgeries than any other hospital in the state. "The culture is also part of it. We treat patients, families and employees with respect."

Sister Marianna also noted that the presence of Kaiser Permanente was a factor. "We are forced into getting out our lab test results faster; therefore, physicians can treat people more quickly. Also, there may be more consistency in the practice patterns of physicians here because of the influence of one large medical group — CPMG."

She added that MedisGroups has sent teams to SJH on four different occasions to study how it achieves its results. Saint Joseph was one of four MedisGroups benchmark hospitals in the U. S.

Relationship Between Kaiser Permanente and Saint Joseph Hospital

LeRoy Sides, MD, who had been with the hospital for many years, noted that when Sister Mary Andrew, the former CEO of Saint Joseph Hospital, brought the original proposal for the Kaiser Permanente affiliation to the hospital's medical staff in 1969, it was rejected. "But Sister Mary Andrew had her heart set on this contract, and the medical staff changed its position. Part of the reason was that Sister wanted to head off the possibility of another hospital's being built in Denver. She knew the community didn't need it."

Dr. Cole said, "We have always approached Saint Joseph Hospital as a partner. We have both worked diligently to make this relationship successful." Chris Binkley added, "We could probably buy beds cheaper by purchasing excess capacity in some of the other hospitals in the area. However, we believe in continuous quality improvement, and part of that philosophy is to find partners you can work with rather than shopping around for the lowest prices."

Relationships among Permanente and independent physicians. One of the SJH board members said that the relationship between independent and CPMG physicians has improved substantially over the past two or three years. "One of the best indicators of this is that our next president of the medical staff will be a Permanente physician; this will be a first."

Several individuals interviewed said that there have been periods of time when the relationships between independent physicians and the Permanente doctors were rocky. However, the key has been the recognition by independent physicians that many Permanente doctors are talented physicians. Of course, many of the interns at SJH have ended up with CPMG; most of these individuals were well known and respected by the independent physicians during their training.

In 1993, many Permanente physicians were active on departmental committees and participated in all medical staff activities.

Negotiating the KP contract. Dennis Wilson said there were serious negotiations with Kaiser Permanente in 1985 at the time the HMO made the decision not to build its own hospital. At that time, Kaiser Permanente represented one-third of the inpatient volume of Saint Joseph Hospital.

According to Wilson, the last go-round of negotiations was conducted by a team of five persons from each organization. One of the major points negotiated was what Kaiser Permanente would pay for, and what the HMO would not pay. Wilson said that the negotiations were open and friendly. "We open our books to them; there are no secrets."

Joint planning. According to Beverly Schulman, Vice President for Planning and Marketing, Kaiser Permanente and SJH have been holding joint planning meetings for the past two years. Individuals involved included the top administrators of both organizations. She added, "The chief financial officers of the two organizations have developed a solid relationship and are able to work out pricing and payment issues that arise."

One point of contention that emerged between the two organizations was KP's decision to build and operate its own outpatient surgery facility. According to one SJH administrator, this had an adverse affect on the volume of the Saint Joseph facility.

Saint Joseph Hospital's Other Physician-Hospital Initiatives

Sister Marianna Bauder said that Saint Joseph Hospital had a policy of working with all of its physicians, and it did this through support of three organizations and the development of a new primary care initiative. She referred to this as a "pluralistic approach."

Robert Collins said there is a need for alternatives in terms of caring for the health care needs of the population. "We need to continue to encourage creativity and experimentation in the way we care for patients. At Saint Joseph Hospital, we are involved in a number of different organizational approaches, and we think this is appropriate."

Medwest. Established in 1985, Medwest was a for-profit, physician-hospital organization created primarily to develop managed care contracts and to provide other services (e.g., billing, computer linkages with professional corporations) for a group of private practice physicians. Medwest was jointly owned by a group of physicians and Saint Joseph Hospital.

In 1993, Medwest had approximately 200 participating physicians; 26 were in primary care. The staff included a CEO and five full-time equivalent employees.

Gregory Ippen, MD and chairman of the board of Medwest, noted that there were 12 members of the medical group board — six primary care physicians and six specialists. Medwest was funded by a percentage of the collections of participating medical practices. Primary care physicians paid 1.5 percent of their collections on contracts arranged through Medwest, and specialists paid 7.0 percent of their collections resulting on contracts with Medwest.

Saint Joseph contributed to Medwest's funding through the purchase of services, including half the cost of supporting The Healthcare Initiative (THI). The total amount paid to Medwest by SJH approximated $400,000 annually.

Dr. Boline, a pathologist, has been a part of Medwest for many years. He said, "It started with an emphasis on primary care and the gatekeeper function, and this is still something we want. Even the specialists in Medwest would agree that we need to beef up primary care."

Key Care. Key Care, established in 1979 as an "Organization of Independent Physicians," was a PPO; it did not engage in capitated or risk contracts. Key Care had approximately 200 physicians, all specialists. Approximately 65 percent of the Key Care physicians were also members of Medwest.

Dr. Sides, the founder of Key Care, remained active in its affairs. He said that Sister Mary Andrew, the former CEO of Saint Joseph, was involved in the formation of the organization. Several of the original contracts were with union trusts, and these continued to represent a significant portion of the PPO arrangements for the organization.

Key Care was a for-profit organization with 15 board members. The staff included an executive director and one part-time employee. Dues were $125 per year for each participating physician. Saint Joseph Hospital paid the salary of the executive director and in return received human resources services from Key Care. The total amount paid by SJH approximated $100,000 annually.

Accord Medical Centers. As mentioned earlier, Accord was the largest multispecialty medical group in the Denver Area. Saint Joseph Hospital, along with Swedish Medical Center, was a financial supporter of Accord. According to Dennis Wilson, Accord continued to experience operating losses. Saint Joseph advanced Accord $3 million in loans, primarily to enable the clinic's move into new space.

Primary care network development. According to Sister Marianna Bauder, SJH recognized the need to continue to build its primary care network and had hired two family practice and three internal medicine physicians and placed them in a southeast Denver location. She referred to this as a primary care "pod." Additional primary care pods were planned. "Most of our primary care physicians are officed near the hospital; we need better geographic distribution." She added, "We have 19 family practice residents, and we need places for them to practice."

Other Aspects of Kaiser Permanente and Saint Joseph Hospital

Information systems development. Chris Binkley said that KP is making huge investments in terms of integrating its clinical and management information systems. According to Ben Chao, Information Services Director, Kaiser Permanente had four strategies for its information system:

- Converting all non-California regions into a common KP system.

- Improving clinical information systems. Chao said that the present information system was stronger in financial data than in clinical information.

- Outcomes analysis. KP began collecting outcomes data in late 1991, and has been sharing the results with physicians. However, the amount of outcomes information will be increased.

- Fully-automated medical records system. When this part of the system becomes operational, physicians will be able order prescriptions and obtain patient demographic information on an on-line basis.

According to Chao, KP invested close to two percent of revenues to expand its information system and another two percent to maintain the current system. "But, the amount will be higher over the next few years, mainly because of the new medical records system."

With this substantial investment in information systems, KP expects to realize some savings in other areas. For example, in 1993, KP had 110 full-time equivalent employees (FTE) assigned to maintaining medical records. According to Chris Binkley, "The investment in clinical information systems would automate most of this work and obviate the need for most of these FTEs."

Scott Waldrop, Vice President and Chief Information Officer for Saint Joseph, said that KP and the hospital have linked some areas of their information systems. "Both of us chose the same vendor for our surgery scheduling system. We are currently selecting a common vendor for linking up the information systems for the laboratory; this will be up and running in a year or so. Our purpose is to share lab results and to allow physicians to track the status of a patient's lab work."

Waldrop said that both KP and the hospital were interested in developing a clinical system. "The vendor selection process will be carried out concurrently once the project progresses to that point."

Corporate culture. Dr. Boline, a member of the SJH board, said that the presence of Permanente physicians has influenced the independent physicians in terms of their thinking more about cost effectiveness. He said, "The Permanente physicians are more management oriented; many of them have received management training, and it shows in the way they think."

Saint Joseph Hospital was also committed to a residency program and to the training of new physicians. There were typically 100 residents at the hospital. According to Dr. Boline, the Permanente physicians made a special effort to work with residents and carry more than their share of the training load.

In terms of how medical practice at KP differs from independent practice, Dr. Cole said, "Our physicians typically do a lot more on the phone. They don't gain anything from having a patient come in personally when it probably isn't necessary."

He went on, "One of the unique aspects of the CPMG culture is the emphasis on cost-effective medicine, and the belief that high quality usually is associated with lower costs. This has been part of our culture for more than two decades, and it is a firmly held belief by our 400 doctors."

Other than Dr. Cole and his three associate medical directors, all physician-administrators within the CPMG practiced medicine at least 50 percent of the time. The associate medical directors spent 20 percent of their time practicing medicine.

Major Accomplishments

This sub-section focuses on the payoffs of the unique relationship between Kaiser Permanente and Saint Joseph Hospital, and on the accomplishments of SJH and its independent physician groups.

The benefits of the Kaiser Permanente and Saint Joseph Hospital relationship. From the hospital's perspective, Robert Collins said that Kaiser Permanente provides a significant volume of patients that "we can count on." Sister Marianna Bauder believes that the Kaiser Permanente approach to practicing medicine has been beneficial for independent physicians and the hospital.

Low-cost providers. As noted earlier, both Kaiser Permanente and Saint Joseph Hospital were the lowest cost providers in the Denver Area. SJH has consistently ranked favorably in terms of average costs per patient day or discharge; this was based on data collected and reported by the Colorado Hospital Association and the State Health Data Commission. Kaiser Permanente was the lowest cost health plan for most Denver Area employers.

On this point, Steve Tomme of KP said that he was concerned about the health plan's ability to retain its competitive edge. "Our competitors are becoming more sophisticated in managing utilization. Look what has happened in southern California where KP is no longer the low-cost health plan."

Sensitivity to the needs of patients. Sanford Zisman, a SJH board member, said that the employees and physicians at SJH were extremely sensitive to the needs of patients. "This relates to the mission of the Sisters of Charity. The Sisters really live it and it rubs off on everyone else."

Quality of care. The accomplishments of SJH in terms of achieving quality outcomes was discussed earlier. Several individuals interviewed attributed a major part of this accomplishment to the presence of the Permanente physicians, and their impact on clinical protocols and a systems approach to practicing medicine.

Ability to centralize inpatient hospitalizations. Steve Tomme of KP said that in his contacts with employers he did not experience resistance to the concept of using one major hospital. "Most of them realize that inpatient hospitalization is an infrequent occurrence. If we hadn't been aggressive in establishing medical offices, this might have been a problem. But, most employers and subscribers are much more concerned about access to their medical office than they are to a hospital."

The economic and quality benefits of concentrating hospital admissions at SJH were discussed previously.

Issues for the Future

Robert Collins, board chairman of SJH, said the organization faced several issues. "One of the top two issues is the need to reconfigure the hospital to make it more in tune with the trend toward outpatient services. Second, the institutional arrangements between the physicians and the hospital, and between physicians and health plans, are going to have to change." He noted that other important issues include confronting the matter of location of the hospital and related facilities, moving ahead with new technology and maintaining economic viability with changes in reimbursement likely to result from health care reform.

Dr. Charles, the chief of the medical staff in 1993, said that he believed that economic credentialing would be forced on the hospital by the pressures of managed care. "Comprecare is already doing it. I don't like the idea of a closed medical staff, but it appears that the pressures on the health care system will force us to move in this direction."

Steven Tomme of KP said that he was concerned that the leveling of prices under health care reform would work against organizations like Kaiser Permanente. "We would lose an important part of our advantage."

Others at KP were concerned about the organization's ability to keep its costs low. There was a general feeling that other HMOs and health plans were improving their management and utilization, and were catching up with KP in terms of narrowing the price differential. However, one person said, "We believe that in the long term we will be successful in managing costs. The benefits of an integrated system have got to pay off."

Finally, there was concern by both KP and Saint Joseph Hospital managers about the need to plan for additional inpatient capacity to accommodate the anticipated growth of the health plan. At the same time, SJH management and its board wanted to keep the hospital open to private practice physicians. Sister Marianna Bauder said, "We have demonstrated that the present system works in terms of low costs and high quality. We think this is advantageous to the community."

* We especially appreciated the help of Chris Binkley, Senior Vice President and Regional Manager for Kaiser Foundation Health Plan of Colorado, and Sister Marianna Bauder, CEO, Saint Joseph Hospital, for making this case study possible.